Lionheart

MATTHEW'S STORY

Katie Ekroth

Orca Book Publishers

"Leaving on a Jet Plane" © 1976, Cherry Lane Music.

Canadian Cataloguing in Publication Data
Ekroth, Katie, 1946-
    Lionheart: Matthew's story

    ISBN 0-920501-50-8
    1. Ekroth, Matthew. 2. Heart — Transplantation
— Patients — British Columbia — Biography. 3.
Lungs — Transplation — Patients — British
Columbia — Biography. 4. Transplantation of
organs, tissues, etc. in children — Biography.
I. Title.
RD598.35.T7E47 1990   362.1'97412'092   C90-091484-X

We gratefully acknowledge the financial support
of the Government of British Columbia.

Publication assistance provided by the Canada Council.

Orca Book Publishers
P.O. Box 5626, Stn. B.
Victoria, B.C. Canada
V8R 6S4

Cover photograph courtesy of *The Vancouver Province*, Colin Savage, photographer.
Cover design by Susan Fergusson.
Printed in Canada

To the countless friends, both known and otherwise,
who in a myriad of ways, became part of Matthew's story.

Special thanks are due to:

Claudette Reed Upton and Trudy Lancelyn — for preparing the manuscript and for their sensitive, caring editorial work.

And to my husband, Don, for his unfailing encouragement. Without his help, this book would never have been completed.

Most of the people in Matthew's story have opted to keep their own names. Others have preferred not to be identified; this wish has been respected.

Preface

I had to write this book.

It started as a compulsion — almost an obsession, in fact. Often throughout Matthew's illness, I would come home from the hospital and scrawl the day's events into a notebook, usually at a feverish pitch. And then at Harefield both Don and I kept diaries which we unloaded into on a daily basis. It was a means both of coping and of remembering, a means of getting things into perspective, of maintaining some sanity. Consequently, when the time came to write this story, detail was easy to come by, as much was already recorded. For the balance, our memories have served us well, and I am also indebted to many of the people involved for their own personal recollections.

On reading through the first draft, the editor laughed at my "cast of thousands."

"You can't mention everyone," she admonished, "and neither can you relate every detail!"

Changes were made with some reluctance, but I've had to learn that she was right.

The book is written largely in the hope of helping to promote organ donor awareness, and to this end I am particularly delighted that Loretta Kane, Senior Transplant Coordinator with the Pacific Organ Retrieval for Transplantation (P.O.R.T.) Program, agreed to contribute to the epilogue.

I am also hopeful that parts of the story may be helpful to others, especially those who struggle daily in their care of a child with catastrophic illness.

And last, but certainly not least, the book is written as a tribute to Matthew — and to acknowledge his spirit and courage. For he truly was a Lionheart!

Lionheart

Chapter One

There is probably no more important job in the world than raising children, nor one for which I was less prepared. It had never occurred to me that I would have any trouble at all being a parent. I sailed into it with all the naïve optimism I'd brought to Canada nine years earlier — not planning overly much, but confident that everything would work out well.

In April 1969, armed with a trunk, two suitcases and my nursing training, I left my native England for the distant shores of Canada. Just for a year, you understand. One of the things that had attracted me to nursing was that it's a universal skill, an ideal career to combine with travel.

I fell in love with the rugged beauty and space of Canada, not to mention the unexpected leap in salary and standard of living. British to the core, I decided that I would just have to sing Rule Britannia from afar. In the summer of 1976, I married a tall, dark and handsome Canadian I had met on a blind date five years earlier. We settled in Vancouver, where Don was already established as a commercial fisherman.

Elizabeth was delivered by emergency cesarean section on January 19, 1978. I learned then that the intensity of the love that a mother has for her child can never be adequately described. It simply has to be experienced.

Matthew was born nineteen months later on August 20, 1979. He, too, was born by C-section, but this time it was elective. No labour, no pain, no fatigue. Don wore his best suit. I still remember the joy; our cup overflowed.

Our pampered golden Labrador, Thor, groaned at the arrival of another intruder. His nose had been put out of joint severely when Elizabeth had arrived and he was ousted to second place. I'm sure he sensed that a further demotion was imminent.

Matthew, like Elizabeth, was a model baby. He slept and fed, fed and slept, and as soon as the development books would allow, he cooed and smiled amiably from one end of the day to the other. Elizabeth, in the meantime, edging closer to the "terrible twos," revved into high gear, and became extraordinarily "busy."

I can see her even now, running from one object to another, touching, smelling, tasting — so much to do and, seemingly, not enough time in which to do it. Twiddling TV knobs, bouncing on Thor, floating blocks in the toilet, playing house in the fireplace cinders, she raced from one adventure to the next like a whirling dervish. It never failed to amaze me just how much this blond, angelic child could accomplish in a day. By suppertime I was always exhausted, which was unfortunate, because supper brought a whole new set of challenges: apple juice on the floor, baked beans in her hair, ice cream up to her elbows. I was often tempted just to hose down the kitchen and my little friend, too.

With no previous experience of babysitting or raising young children, I didn't realize that Elizabeth had leapt the boundaries of normal two-year-old behaviour. It was, in fact, a whole year later before the word "hyperactive" crept into my vocabulary. I learned that magic could be spun simply with substitutions in her diet.

Matthew, in the meantime, would be sitting in his baby-seat, or springing about in the Jolly Jumper, smiling agreeably and following all the frenzied activity with bright, inquisitive eyes. "Don't go getting any ideas, little fella," I'd warn.

The Jolly Jumper, that marvellous invention that has launched millions of toddlers, had again done a remarkable job. Matthew's legs were sturdy and strong; he could outrun me anytime. Motherhood was proving to be a most challenging career. I often thought back wistfully to my days in nursing. Twelve-hour shifts in Emergency were a piece of cake compared to this!

We moved in the spring of 1981, when Elizabeth was three years old and Matthew twenty months. It took two hours — well, maybe three — for us to feel at home in Tsawwassen. Nestled between the ocean, the Canada-US border, and the fertile farmland of the Fraser River delta, this little community — then with a population of about 16,000 — is very self-reliant. Within a few blocks are shopping, beaches, schools, walking paths, ice rink, bowling alley, swimming pool, library — in fact, every amenity. Tsawwassen is only twenty miles from Vancouver, yet somehow misses much of the rain that city is famous for. Don kept his gillnet fishing boat, the *Sunburst*, at a nearby dock. We couldn't think of a more ideal place to bring up our children.

And best of all I found a babysitting co-op. Yes, indeed, every amenity. I now had a ready-made network of other mothers of young children to rely on for advice and moral support, and an outlet for the hellbent-for-leather energy of our two little ones. We had the world by the tail — a blissful marriage, two precious children, a lovely house in an idyllic setting.

Days, months and years run together, but certain moments stand out clear and true, undiminished by time. When we cast back in our memories, it's often the thinnest slices of time we remember, single moments with the force to define an entire year. For me, March 17, 1982, is one such day.

I've often thought back to that day. Was there any warning? Any premonition that we were singled out for the traumatic fight to save a child's life? There were none.

In fact, I recall basking in the warm spring sunshine, feeling the renewal of hope and the satisfaction that comes with the knowledge that one can survive life's dark days — the feeling that, if anything, we had already paid our price for happiness. Three months earlier, on December 6, 1981, I had given birth to a stillborn baby boy. Knowing before the birth that he had died did nothing to alleviate my sense of pain and loss.

Late in November, seven months into the pregnancy, I had suddenly become aware that the frequent movements in my rapidly expanding belly had stopped. I was only mildly concerned. Problems with a pregnancy at this late stage were rare. The baby was sleeping, I reasoned, just enjoying a few quiet days.

On the fourth day of this new development I went down to the medical clinic. Fear had nudged me into action, but I was still nonchalant. I stammered apologies to the nurse/receptionist for being a bother. I had been in just a week earlier for a routine maternity check, and both the baby and I had passed with flying colours. Dr. Martin listened intently while I explained the baby's sudden change in activity. "It's probably nothing, but I need reassurance," I told him.

As part of my nursing training, I had taken a three-month obstetrics course. I had listened many times to the heartbeat of the new life growing within the mother. With practice, there is usually no problem locating the rapid thump-thump, thump-thump. Why then, was Dr. Martin taking so long? He exchanged the stethoscope for a more sensitive fetal monitor. I held my breath. An eternity passed. He finally raised his head.

"Well, I can hear some heart sounds, but it's hard to know whether they're yours or the baby's. I think you should have a scan just to be on the safe side." His face was grave, but I chose to be hopeful. Anything else was unthinkable. The nurse asked me to wait while she phoned the Willow Pavilion at Vancouver General Hospital.

My mind wandered back to my nursing days and in particular to the patients I had cared for on the gynaecology wards. I thought of the many women who had lost their babies at various stages of development. I had prided myself on being a good nurse. My rooms were kept tidy, beds made, medications given on time and notes kept carefully up to date. I realized now that I had failed these patients. I had had no knowledge of the complex emotional machinery that comes into play when a miscarriage or stillbirth occurs. I had never heard of bonding, let alone comprehended the love that a mother feels for her developing child. Neither had I entertained the idea that a mother could grieve for a baby she had never known. After all, she could always try again, and replace that baby with another. How little I knew then! How much I now understood!

Don picked me up at the doctor's office and we drove the twenty miles to the hospital. In the back of the car, uncommonly quiet, sat Elizabeth who was almost four, and Matthew, who had turned two in August.

"Why is your face red, Mommy?" Elizabeth asked. I couldn't stop crying.

The young medical technician made small talk about the coming Christmas season while he conducted the scan. Keeping perfectly still, as if good behaviour could sway the results in my favour, I searched his face for clues.

A nurse returned to check our progress. The young man spoke without looking up. "I can't pick up the whole picture. I'm going to take Mrs. Ekroth and have a better look with the big scanner." He pointed at parts of the strange picture on the screen and the nurse nodded in agreement. I knew then, without any doubt, that our baby had died. What had I done wrong? How could this possibly have happened? I had read all the books on producing healthy babies. Cottage cheese, liver and spinach had become my staple diet. I had never smoked or taken medication. I had drunk only the odd small glass of wine — surely that couldn't have killed our child.

The nurse, now serious and protective, led me down to the busy room where a big scanner performed its perfunctory task of documenting the death of our child. The technician and a doctor examined the irregular pictures. The doctor shook her head, perhaps trying to warn me, trying to buy more time.

"I'm sorry," she said finally. "Your baby has died. We've estimated that it happened about four days ago. I'm afraid we can't tell why from our scans. I'm so sorry."

Raw nerve endings relayed messages of overwhelming sadness to my brain, my heart, every inch of me. There was nothing to do but weep. I would never know this child. Never hold him or kiss him. Never feel the warm softness of his cheek against mine. The choosing of names had been but an exercise. The new stroller would carry only Teddy-Ann or a favourite doll. The anticipation had been merely a fantasy. There would be no baby.

That evening Don phoned shocked relatives and friends. Everyone was stunned, of course. Pregnancies were vulnerable at three and four months. Seven months was safe — everyone knew that. Even premature babies could survive at this late stage. It was outrageous. In this first year in Tsawwassen we had formed strong bonds with our friends in the babysitting co-op. There were flowers, cards, attempts at saying the right words. And sometimes, no contact for fear of saying the wrong ones.

The obvious comforter was that we already had two healthy children. Indeed, it was a comfort, but it also belittled our loss, and made me feel even more protective of the dead baby. The truth is that — apart from a simple "I'm sorry" — there are no right words.

"Mommy not cry." Little Matthew's big blue eyes looked into mine. At two years old he still had a baby's plump cheeks. His eyes were framed in long dark lashes and his soft brown hair curled at the ends. He climbed onto my knee and put his little arms around my neck. No one hugged quite like Matthew. I felt he was too young to know of our loss. "Mommy sick," I told him.

That simple explanation could not suffice for Elizabeth. For the past three months she had shared in our excitement and anticipation. She had placed her small, grubby hand on my tummy many times and felt the vigorous movements of the life inside. She had practised pushing the stroller in anticipation of long walks with the baby. She had listened intently as we discussed the impending birth and all the ways in which she could help once the baby was home. And now she would have to be told that there would be no baby, after all.

Don set her petite frame on his knee. He chose his words with care.

"Do you remember, Elizabeth, the birds' eggs that we found out under the tree last spring?"

"I 'member," she said, her blond head nodding up and down.

"Do you remember the special one? — the one with the little bird still inside?"

"Yes," she said, her blue eyes searching his face.

"Well, remember, even though the mama and the papa bird loved it dearly and cared for it as best they could, that egg and its baby, for some reason, died. Do you remember how sad it made us feel?" The blond head nodded again, this time more slowly.

Don hugged his small daughter close.

"You know that Mommy has a baby inside of her tummy, don't you? You've seen it grow and felt it move."

"Mommy says I can help her with the baby . . ." The voice is quieter than usual.

"Well," Don continued, intent on staying on track, "for some reason, that baby has died, just like the little bird. Mom and I tried very hard, but something went wrong. It's all a part of nature, isn't it, like the baby bird."

"But the baby'll get better." It is more a statement than a question.

"Did the little bird get better?"

Elizabeth sat quietly for what seemed like a long, long time. She reached over and pulled her friend Blanket from where it lay on the bed. She hugged it to her closely, chewing on one ragged corner. At barely four years old, she was learning a sobering truth: parents can't always make everything right. They don't have complete control. She clambered down from Don's knee and turned to face him.

"Will we bury it in the garden too?" she asked.

Dr. Martin referred me to an obstetrician, Dr. Ann Kendall. No one could have been more gentle or shown more empathy than she. There was no easy way to deal with the situation. I had been automatically booked to have this baby delivered by cesarean the coming February. Since the baby had died, I imagined I would undergo the C-section immediately.

I was horrified to learn that this wouldn't be the case. Apparently, there's too much risk of complications and infection to deliver a dead baby this way. Modern medicine's only safe option is to induce labour by administering drugs intravenously, and allow the baby to be delivered naturally, through the birth canal. The very thought appalled me. To go through the pains of labour only to deliver a dead child! At least with a C-section I would've been anaesthetized, and not consciously involved either physically or emotionally.

I was admitted to the obstetrics floor at Richmond General Hospital. Fortunately the floor was quiet and I was the only patient in the four-bed room. I had dreaded being with other expectant mothers. How on earth could I tell jubilant mothers-to-be of our tragedy?

"Hello, Mrs. Ekroth."

An attractive nurse, not much older than I, stood by my bed. She wasn't carrying any of the tools of her profession, she had simply come to talk. She told me of her own experience just three years earlier when she, too, had lost a baby late in pregnancy. She had gone into premature labour when she was six months pregnant; her tiny son had no chance of survival. Eight years have passed since this woman shared her story with me, and I don't remember all that was said, but I do remember clearly the comfort in her message: Others have passed this way before. They have survived and gone on, and so will you.

On the morning of Sunday, December 6, Dr. Kendall started the Pitocin drip. Don was with me in the delivery room. "We really have to find other ways to spend our weekends," he joked.

The familiar cramps of childbirth ebbed and flowed, and by late afternoon I was racked by sickening pains. Don encouraged me with my breathing levels, but I was fast losing control. The nurse gave me an injection of Demerol, and then another three hours later. There was no reason to withhold medication, the baby's health not being of concern.

Dr. Kendall hovered, waiting for nature to take its course. In spite of my drug-induced haze, I was aware of the crescendo of muscular activity in my abdomen. A moment later, the baby was born. "The umbilical cord was wrapped around the baby's neck," the doctor said quietly. And then, very gently, "Do you want to know the sex? It's a boy. Do you want to see him? No? Very well. We'll take care of him."

It's unfortunate but true that we can't rehearse for the more important decisions in our lives for I soon knew that the ones I had made that night were wrong. And in light of the events that followed with Matthew, it has come back to haunt me with a vengeance. I had hoped that by treating this loss as a miscarriage I could recover quickly. I wanted to deny that there ever had been a real baby. I didn't want a history of grief and loss. I didn't want to say in answer to "How many children do you have?" that we had two, but had lost a baby. We were a happy family. I wanted no black clouds in our skies.

If I could go back in time to that birth, I would hold that tiny discoloured three-pound body. He would be acknowledged and named. He would have a Christian burial and officially be a part of our family.

It's too late to change these things, but that child is still with me in spirit, and I silently acknowledge him every year on his birthday. Little did we know then how very significant this loss would be in the years to come.

Dr. Elisabeth Kübler-Ross, the eminent pioneer of the emotional mysteries surrounding death and grief, has defined the stages to be expected: denial, shock, anger, guilt, depression. Thankfully, I passed through the first four stages quickly. But, as frequently happens, I then became ensnared by depression, a sensation of almost overwhelming sadness.

December was upon us. There were presents to be bought, decorations to be dusted off and hung, cards to be written, Christmas cookies to be baked. Elizabeth and Matthew needed care and reassurance, but I felt like doing nothing. What mattered any more? I was almost offended that other people carried on cheerfully with the hustle and bustle of the season. Didn't they know that our baby had died? Didn't they care?

I drifted aimlessly through the crowded malls and shops, my pain only magnified by the display of celebration. Angelic choirs piped agonizing renditions of "O Holy Child" and "Away in a Manger." It seemed that nearly every woman was pregnant, and those who weren't were pushing smiling infants in strollers. With presents unbought, I fled back to the sanctuary of home. Don was an enormous help in maintaining some semblance of normalcy for the children. While I grappled with the emotional repercussions of our loss, he grappled with the grocery list, babysitting and laundry. Not being bonded to this baby in the same way as I was, he was better able to remain detached and to deal with the situation rationally.

Winter turned to spring and I was gratefully aware of the healing effects of time.

I had another reason to welcome the warmer weather. Matthew had coughed for most of the winter, a deep, racking cough. Several courses of antibiotics had done little to modify its ominous tone. These winter bugs, how we mothers hate them! Never mind, spring's warm sunshine would chase them away, and with summer close on its heels, we had much to look forward to.

On the morning of March 17, with the tender but restored spirits of one who has been put to the test and has triumphed, I returned to Dr. Martin's office with Matthew. He had just finished another course of antibiotics, but was still coughing. Dr. Martin listened carefully to his chest sounds with a stethoscope, reviewed the growing file and reached for a requisition form.

"This has gone on for five months. Let's get a chest X-ray, just to be on the safe side."

We picked up Elizabeth from pre-school on the way home, and arrived in time for the children to watch the last ten minutes of "Sesame Street." After lunch, I nestled Matthew down into bed for his afternoon nap. His little fingers caressed the satiny side of his snuggy blanket and his best friend Doggy rested on the pillow by his head. Shy elephants smiled down at him from the wallpaper, and he smiled up at me as his heavy lids drooped. He was asleep before I reached the door.

I took a chair from the kitchen and sat on the back patio in the sunshine. Thor lay on the grass close to my feet, basking in the indolence of the day. Elizabeth was darting indoors and out. I thought of Don, away herring fishing. I hoped things were going well.

"Mommy, Dr. Martin's on the phone," Elizabeth called from the kitchen.

"Hello, Dr. Martin." My mind was blank. Totally unsuspecting.

"Hello, Mrs. Ekroth. I'm calling about Matthew's X-rays. I've looked at them with the radiologist and there seems to be a problem. I'd like you to take Matthew to see a Dr. Mirhady, who's a children's specialist. My nurse has already made an appointment. Do you have a pencil handy?"

My mouth went dry and my stomach turned over. I heard my own voice coming from somewhere.

"What kind of problem, Dr. Martin?" How could I sound so calm?

He explained that there appeared to be unusual patterning on Matthew's lungs.

"What kind of patterning?"

Again, he was patient and brief. "We don't know what it is. The patterning is throughout both lungs."

"Do you think it's an infection?" Of course, the perfect explanation. But I sensed that Dr. Martin was uncomfortable. He hesitated, protecting.

"No, it appears to be a chronic problem." The world stopped. Chronic. Our lovable little two-year-old son with a chronic lung condition. There must be some mistake.

"Are you all right, Mrs. Ekroth? Can you manage to do this?"

Again, I heard a voice questioning, hoping against hope for an answer to appease my fear, to explain the abnormalities. "And do you have a diagnosis, Dr. Martin?" My legs were suddenly jelly. I concentrated on self-control.

He was quiet, almost apologetic. "We really can't tell without further tests, but the pictures suggest cystic fibrosis. I'm sorry you have to be worried again."

Cystic fibrosis. To me it was a death sentence. Fifteen years earlier as a student nurse, I had worked in one of the big London hospitals. I well remembered the children with cystic fibrosis. They were desperately thin and pale, and coughed endlessly trying to dislodge the thick secretions invading their lung tissue. And they died; always, they died. As I floundered, shocked and grief-stricken on that March afternoon, I could never have guessed that there would be days to come when even this diagnosis would have been good news.

Chapter Two

When I married Don, I not only acquired a husband, I also acquired a second family. Don's parents, sister Lonnie, brother Lorne, and their spouses and children all lived within a ten-mile radius of us. And they truly were a close family. No grapevine ever worked more efficiently. Good news was conveyed with great speed from one unit to another so that all could celebrate. Any dispute would rumble from phone to phone, or bear dissection over bottomless mugs of coffee. And during bad times, everyone would be there. Above all else, the bad times were to be shared.

"Your face is red again! Who're you phoning, Mommy?" Elizabeth had picked up that something was wrong, and, like a homing pigeon, sensed that the kitchen was the place to be.

"I'm phoning Gramma, dear," I told her, sidestepping her initial comment. Don's mother listened in horrified silence as, between sobs, I described the events of the day.

"Oh, Katie, this is terrible. But don't you worry now. It's going to be all right. Now, Don won't be home from fishing for at least a week. You just bundle yourself and the children over here. And bring Thor. You can all stay with Gramma."

Mom took charge. Thank God. I couldn't seem to function. Fear attacked from every side. I prayed a short prayer that God would make it all right. But God wasn't there. Just a void, emptiness, nothing. I washed my face and pulled myself together.

Steeling myself, I crept into Matthew's room and looked down at our sleeping child. "Please God, make him well," I whispered. But again, there was nothing. No reassurance, no hint of peace.

I had never known God well. As young children, we attended church with my father every Sunday morning while my mother stayed home to cook our big Sunday lunch — typically roast beef with Yorkshire pudding, gravy, potatoes and vegetables. Sadly, almost a lost tradition.

The church was historically magnificent, having held the place of honour overlooking the village green for more than seven hundred years. The wooden pews were beautifully engraved — but very hard. Like many of England's churches, it was built of stone and damply cold inside. The service, in language difficult to understand, seemed to go on forever. All my memories are of dull sermons to mostly empty pews; all in all, not exactly a springboard to spiritual bliss.

As we grew older, we were allowed to attend evensong. By this time I had developed acne and a painful crush on one of the local farmers' sons. I never missed a service, my only opportunity to glimpse my uncaring blond Adonis. Needless to say, my spiritual life benefited little from this exercise in unrequited love. From then on, there were smatterings of religion. Black stockings catching on the wooden floors as we knelt to pray, morning and night, in the long, thirty-bed hospital wards in London. Hope that God was listening as one particularly unpleasant nursing tutor prayed for "all evils of this night to be removed." The magic of a Christmas Eve candlelight service. Religion was something to take or leave as suited the mood. Mostly, it suited me to leave it, and bring it out on the occasional Sunday, and, of course, on Christmas and Easter. But that was all.

When Elizabeth and Matthew were born, I dusted off my spiritual file. I did, after all, want our children to grow up with a healthy system of values. At that point, I returned to church, recognizing Sunday school as a positive experience for children. I wanted our children to be good, kind, obedient and loving, and these teachings are, of course, reinforced in the church environment.

On moving to Tsawwassen, I sought out the United Church, housed in a lovely new building and boasting an excellent choir. The Sunday school was active and continually in need of helpers. It was a good place for me to start. The pre-schoolers were just my level: no one was likely to ask me to expound on Ecclesiastes, and I was as skilled as I needed to be with glue, crayons and action songs.

Matthew was very comfortable praying. His concentration focused entirely on the subject at hand.

"Would you please say grace today, Matthew?" His eyes would close tightly as he clasped his hands together.

"Dear Jesus. Thank you for this day. Thank you for my friends. Thank you for my family. Please help me to understand that You are always with us. Thank you for my bed. Thank you for Transformers . . ." Skin would be forming on the gravy.

His bedtime prayers were the same. And his hugs were warmth and love. I looked down on him now, hoping against hope that his faith and rapport with God could do what mine could not.

Mom was waiting at the door when we arrived around suppertime. The family had been alerted and were all on hand. The mere sight of them was enough to start my carefully suppressed weeping all over again. ''You don't have to cry, Mommy,'' Matthew comforted. Much to my horror, I found I had difficulty looking him in the eye; my natural instinct to protect him was in conflict with my need to protect myself.

The following afternoon Lonnie's husband, Bill, drove Matthew and me into Vancouver for our appointment with Dr. Mirhady, the paediatrician. Hope had, of necessity, entwined itself around my fear. Dr. Mirhady would have some simple explanation. We'd all be laughing with relief around the supper table tonight.

Dr. Mirhady, now past middle age, is a quiet, methodical, conscientious expert in childhood illness. I had the distinct impression that he had seen it all, and that he missed nothing. Even as he questioned me, attempting to form a picture of Matthew's medical history, his eyes never left the little boy. Sherlock Holmes couldn't have competed with his subtle detective work. And then a detailed repeat of Dr. Martin's examination — weight, temperature, body measurements, blood pressure, chest sounds, percussion, mouth, nose and ears, all checked and rechecked. And finally, the scrutiny completed, a full written history. Nothing was overlooked.

Dr. Mirhady broke the silence.

''Well, Matthew, when your mommy has helped you to dress again, you can go and see which toys you'd like to play with in the waiting room.''

It was now my turn. Fear returned in full force. Dr. Mirhady carefully, methodically, placed the papers in the folder and put down his pen. He spoke slowly.

He admitted that he was very puzzled. The patterning on the X-ray was diffuse and roughly symmetrical. It was possibly caused by low-grade chest infections due to a deficiency in the immune system. Blood tests would eliminate a number of other possibilities, but they weren't real probabilities.

No, on the present findings, his opinion concurred with that of the radiologist. The most likely diagnosis, the one to rule out first, was cystic fibrosis. The piece of the puzzle that didn't fit was that cystic fibrosis is a disease in which digestion is also impaired. Its victims fail to thrive, remaining thin and pale. Matthew, on the other hand, was sturdy and stocky with plump, rosy cheeks. He didn't fit the typical picture at all. I was being thrown a lifeline. Over the next five years we were to become well acquainted with the essential crutch that goes by the name of Hope. Now, however, I didn't trust myself to speak.

Dr. Mirhady continued. He quietly explained that medical science has made progress with cystic fibrosis. Many patients now live to young adulthood, and there is, of course, the constant hope of a cure being found. In the meantime, however, it would be wise to keep Matthew away from other children as much as possible, to prevent future chest infections.

So, there was to be no reprieve. We Anglo-Saxons are well trained, are we not, in the art of self-control? I desperately wanted to sob, protest, kick, scream. Instead: "Thank you, Dr. Mirhady. We'll be in touch after the tests."

Supper that evening was a sombre affair. I searched for answers. Why Matthew? Why us? Indeed, why us again? Had I done something wrong during the pregnancy? Had I inadvertently harmed this little boy even as he was developing? Was God punishing me? Was he tired of my complacency? Why were we being singled out for such unwelcome attention? No answers came. Mom, Pop, Lonnie and Bill tried to buoy me up. Numbed themselves, they delved for reasonable explanations. The most acceptable, and the one that I clung to, was that Matthew was merely demonstrating an unusual form of the allergies and asthma that plagued the Ekroth side of the family. Temporarily reassured, we all agreed that he'd soon grow out of it, and live to a ripe old age.

Mom needed to cover all the bases. "And anyway, Katie," she said, "even if it should be something more serious, the way the world's going, we'll all be blown up by a nuclear bomb long before Matthew has any real problems." In some inexplicable way, I found this to be a most comforting thought.

There was an important decision to be made. Don was away on the fishing grounds waiting, along with hundreds of others, for the herring to be ready for harvesting. Thousands upon thousands of the silver and black bodies move in and out of the shallows, while the fishermen wait for the word to be given. When "shaking" begins, the activity is frenetic, for fortunes can be made within days. Should I be upsetting Don at this crucial point of the season?

I wasn't capable of making the decision myself, but Lonnie and Mom concluded that no purpose would be served by alarming him at this stage. First, there was no absolute diagnosis; and second, what could he do anyway? It would be madness for him to desert our enormous investment in the fishing and return home. So when Don phoned from the boat the following morning, having tracked us down at his parents' place, I said nothing about the threat to Matthew's life.

That afternoon Bill again drove Matthew and me into Vancouver. This time our destination was B.C. Children's Hospital. Matthew was booked for the "sweat test," a simple and effective means of testing for cystic fibrosis. The lab technician also took a blood specimen for full blood work, punctuated by much crying and screaming — there's no easy way to take blood from an alert two-year-old. And then, back to Mom's to resume the waiting and worrying.

Two days later in the afternoon, Lonnie answered the phone. I was in the bathroom down the hall, but I could hear her jubilant shout, "Oh, that's wonderful!" And then, with her hand clasped over the mouthpiece, "Katie, the sweat test was negative."

Oh, the relief, the indescribable relief. A reprieve of momentous proportions. A millstone removed. "Thank you, Lord, thank you," I whispered to my elusive acquaintance. The bush telegraph was soon in action. The good news spread like wildfire through our network of friends. But even as we laughed and hugged each other, we couldn't ignore the deep and ominous coughing that permeated our celebrations.

Dr. Mirhady was perplexed. Very perplexed. And, he assured us, he wasn't alone — every radiologist he knew had pondered over Matthew's chest X-rays. Any suggested diagnosis had already been eliminated by the sweat test and blood work. Nothing, apart from the X-ray itself, appeared abnormal. It was all very intriguing. Don and I felt that we, too, would have been intrigued if he weren't our own child.

A few weeks later, the chilling, racking cough ceased as if by magic. Perhaps this nightmare would pass after all. Matthew was gaining in size and strength each day. His round cheeks were rosy and his big blue eyes sparkled with mischief. Dr. Mirhady referred Matthew on to Dr. Gordon Pirie, a specialist in both paediatrics and chest diseases. Again, the thorough history and examination. Again, no answers. Dr. Pirie told us that the next step in diagnosis normally would be to admit Matthew to Children's Hospital and perform a lung biopsy under anaesthetic. The procedure carried serious risks with it, and since Matthew was so well, it would be inappropriate at this stage. Much heartened, we agreed entirely.

Don and I tried to put our fears behind us and think positive thoughts. I bought each of the children a large bottle of vitamins. It was marvellous to have a small measure of control again. As the days, weeks and months passed without any setbacks or recurrences of the cough, our hopes soared and our confidence for the future returned.

Spring turned into summer, and the children grew and thrived. I took care to keep Matthew away from other children as much as possible, as Dr. Mirhady had suggested, to prevent his picking up colds and coughs.

It wasn't easy. He was growing into a very sociable youngster and didn't appreciate being isolated from his friends. He was also very physically coordinated. Cartwheels and flips were his specialty. There was nothing and nowhere that he could not climb. One day I answered the phone to hear extreme urgency in the normally calm voice of my friend and neighbour, Eleanor Fowler.

"Katie, I thought you'd like to know that Matthew's climbing out of his bedroom onto the carport roof." Eleanor could see his antics from her kitchen window across the road. I raced up the stairs, and dragging him in by the scruff of his neck, punctuated the mandatory lecture with a sound smack on the bottom.

Like many other moms and pre-schoolers, we spent hours in the various parks around our area. Swings, tires, poles and slides became Matthew's substitute for playmates. I would sometimes take the chance and leave him at one of the co-op moms' houses, but only after a probing exchange on the health of the other children.

The cooler days of autumn were soon upon us. Smiling mothers were everywhere, carrying on the annual September conversations.

"Yes, a lovely summer, thanks, but I'm ready for a change."

"They're short a Brownie leader. I should offer, but..."

"Now that she's in school, I'd like to go back to work again."

Elizabeth was enroled in pre-school and Matthew would normally have started, too. He had turned three in August, and it would have been an excellent chance to practise socializing and sharing. He needed that opportunity. He was interested in everything and was more than ready to learn at that level, but the risks were too great. Likewise, he could not join the pre-school class at Sunday school. He stayed home with Don while Elizabeth and I left for church in our finery. The same applied to parties, unless, of course, they were very small and I was able to monitor the presence of any offending dripping noses.

At the end of October, the babysitting co-op organized a big Halloween party. Elizabeth dressed as Raggedy Ann, and Don, in a unique interpretation of Little Red Riding Hood, accompanied her. When I tell you that Don is six-foot-two and sports a mustache, you can imagine how funny he looked in pigtails and large red cloak with his little basket over his arm. Not wanting to frustrate our young son further, I spent the entire afternoon with him away from home, so he wasn't even aware that he had missed out on yet another event.

His days revolved around "Sesame Street" and "Mr. Rogers" and outings with me. He spent hours on his bike and in other physical pursuits. Gymnastics was his favourite, and sometimes we'd kick a soccer ball around, or try our hands at a modified game of tennis. He had very few breaks from me, or I from him. Much to my distress, I realized that our once loving, cuddly, sweet-natured son was becoming increasingly aggressive and rebellious. He and Elizabeth fought and argued endlessly, and neither of them displayed the compliance and obedience that I had assumed would be there for the asking. I had planned to raise happy, well-behaved children. What had gone wrong? How could I possibly have lost control so soon? Confidence in my parenting abilities was shattered. I felt totally inadequate.

I was unaware at the time that parents everywhere were facing exactly the same feelings of bewildered powerlessness.

"I'd never have dared to talk to my father like that."

"I wouldn't have dreamed of disobeying my mother."

My own upbringing, while happy and traditional, had given me few tools for raising my own children. I was the fifth daughter of six children. My father was the only doctor in our village, so he was never off-duty, and my mother, a trained nurse, was equally busy. She helped him in his practice and ran the house as well. With little in the way of packaged entertainment available, we learned to amuse ourselves. We'd spend hours playing two-ball and hide-and-seek, or going for long country walks. My memory's far from perfect, but it seems to me that we did what we were told, when we were told. There was never any back-chat — it simply wasn't tolerated. It was still the era when children were to be seen but not heard, and no one ever questioned it. Compliance was the name of the game. It was a very different world from the one into which my children were born.

What had changed? My troubled searchings at the public library unearthed *Children: The Challenge* by Rudolf Dreikurs — and along with it, some answers. The structure of society, and consequently the family, has changed. In the more traditional patriarchal order, the man was the head of the family, the wife was second, and the children were "low men on the totem pole." Everyone knew his or her place. All behaviours and expectations were established by tradition. The children, as inferior beings, did as their superiors asked. However, this autocratic system has become a democratic system, aided mainly by the women's movement.

"Women proclaimed their equality with men; and as the husband lost his power over his wife, both parents lost their power over the children," Dreikurs says. I could understand and relate to this in the light of my own experience. We're living in a time when not only do children need to be trained, but parents need to learn how to train them. The rules have all changed. We buy self-help books, and flock in droves to parenting classes, to master what to say to our children and how to say it. The whole subject embraces an entirely new language: positive parental attitudes, your child's self-esteem. It sounds like serious business, and indeed it is.

Unfortunately, our son seemed to learn faster than we did, and our newly acquired skills were frequently challenged in some totally unexpected and subtle manner. Consistency is a challenge any time; for parents, it can be near to impossible.

On one of our recheck visits to Dr. Mirhady, I poured out my problems of living with an exuberant three-year-old who was unable to use the customary methods of letting off steam.

"Put a metal bar in the back garden and have him play on that," he advised, smiling benignly. I didn't like to tell this kind gentleman that Matthew had already mastered the carport roof, and was now seeking bigger thrills.

In January, Don and I decided to start cautiously integrating Matthew into some activities. We chose ice skating lessons and a Tiny Tot tumbling course — both of which, we reasoned, were held in large airy buildings, and would require minimal close contact with other children.

The ice skating was a failure. He got cold, fell frequently, and experienced renewed frustration at owning a mother who wouldn't let him buy junk food from the vending machine. But the tumbling course worked wonders. It was something at which he could excel. Not only could he expend some of his pent-up energy, he could also socialize and, in the words of the child-raising manuals, "build self-esteem." It was a step in the right direction.

A second big step came in April. My friend Geraldine was well aware of my fears and problems of the past year. Matthew frequently played with her small son, Robert, so she had had ample opportunity to witness his frustrations first-hand. She knew of an excellent play-group and wondered if it might help. Sherry, its manager, was gentle but firm, and believed in giving much personal attention to the children. Thus it was that Sherry's Place came to be Matthew's big weekly outing. We armed Sherry with the mysteries of his medical history, and she joined the expanding group of Tsawwassen mothers on the lookout for infections.

Matthew blossomed. This was his "school," his friends, his independence. He was getting to go places after all.

It was now just over a year since the first terrifying X-ray. I had almost convinced myself that the danger was past. Whatever the problem was, he would grow out of it. A further X-ray at this time presented exactly the same picture — no better, no worse. Dr. Mirhady observed Matthew and then the X-rays. He shook his head. "Matthew is a mystery," was all he could say.

In the fall of 1983, Matthew, who had just turned four, started pre-school and was, at last, allowed to fully integrate with other children. He was like an animal suddenly let off the leash. He couldn't get enough of life and the experiences it had to offer. He needed to be at the head of every line-up and the front of every group, and he volunteered eagerly for tasks, always wanting to be first. One of his hardest lessons was that this was neither fair nor possible.

He and his friend Gregory spent hours goading their bikes over jumps on our driveway. They'd recharge their batteries as they drank in the latest televised adventures of He-Man and Transformers, and then they'd be back out playing football, soccer or tennis by the hour. They were such good days.

I have so many memories of these two years, and the overriding feeling is that each day was better than the one before. We seized the opportunity to travel now that the children were a little older. During this precious time, we visited England, Disneyland and Hawaii, enduring adventures both great and small.

On our trip to England, we stayed with my mother in Cheshire. It was a chance for the children to get to know their Granny Petal better and to become well acquainted with her overflowing candy tin. There were also aunts, uncles, cousins and friends of the family to impress and aggravate in equal measure.

Among these family friends, I recall a very pleasant, archetypally English lady who appeared at Mom's door one afternoon. Resplendent in gloves and felt hat, she was the perfect picture of a refined lady prepared to participate in the ritual of afternoon tea. Matthew reached her first. Eyes sparkling, he held out his brand-new plastic handcuffs for the agreeable, unsuspecting lady to survey. Then, faster than she could utter "scones and jam," he had her. She was his prisoner. What a victory! His hoots of laughter brought my mom, sister and me rushing to the hall. It's difficult to shake hands when one is handcuffed, but the stalwart visitor did her best. We nodded pleasantly at each other and found the woman a chair while we all frantically searched for the missing key. The captive could not, of course, drink her tea or eat her scones and jam, but she politely said it didn't matter, insisting, "this sort of thing happens all the time." An urgent, hurried family conference in the kitchen decided that an immediate supper invitation would be appropriate, but the wayward key surfaced in a garbage can at that point, and the nice lady was released to the outside world.

Disneyland is, of course, pure magic, pure pleasure, a little piece of heaven on earth for the child in each of us. We all delighted in "It's a Small World" and the many other rides and shows. The children soaked up the sights and sounds like sponges. Admittedly, some of the sensations were too much for Matthew. When the Caribbean pirate pointed his pistol in our direction, Matt disappeared, shrieking, beneath the seat, and refused to surface until the ride was over.

Universal Studios is another must for visitors to Los Angeles. As we waited to enter the main building, a hostess asked if there were any little boys who would like to volunteer for a special part. Matthew, aided and abetted by his father, was quick to respond, and it transpired that he was to be used as a model to demonstrate some special effects. At the appropriate moment, he clambered up onto a bicycle seat, and, with E.T. balanced in the front basket, he pedalled the stationary bike as fast as his little legs would go. And there, on the screen in front of us, was Matthew, playing the part of Elliott rescuing his friend E.T., in silhouette against the moon.

His moment of glory over, he scrambled down onto the stage amid loud applause and bowed deeply to his audience, quite at home in the limelight. I blinked back tears of maternal pride. It was definitely one of life's finer moments.

In December 1984, we took the children on a two-week Hawaiian holiday. Warmth and sunshine, snorkelling, palm trees and sandcastles, papayas, sunsets, birds of paradise and tropical fish, whales, beachcombing and mai tais — it was everything a tropical holiday should be. When we arrived at Honolulu airport for our return flight we were happy, tanned and relaxed. We were dressed to suit the South Pacific weather and needed to change to warm clothes for our return to the cold Canadian winter. Elizabeth and I headed to the women's restroom, leaving Don and Matthew with the hand luggage. When we emerged ten minutes later, bundled in sweaters, Don's anxious face met us at the door.

"Is he with you?"

"Who?"

"Matthew, of course."

"No, I left him with you."

"Well, he's gone. I can't find him anywhere. I just took my eyes off him for a minute to get our warm clothes from the bag, and when I turned around, he'd gone."

"He can't be far."

Elizabeth sat by our bags in the waiting area, and promised faithfully not to move. Don headed in one direction and I in another. We hunted high and low, and after five minutes met back with Elizabeth. Now it was serious. Panic gripped me. We were both breathing rapidly. Don was pale beneath his tan.

"He's been gone now for nearly fifteen minutes." Don's eyes were dark and scared. Our 747 was due to leave for Vancouver in twenty minutes, but it was no longer important. There would be other flights. We could always get home another way. But where was our son?

What parent doesn't feel a pang on chancing across the latest notice reporting a missing child? Their haunting faces call out to us from milk cartons, newspapers, and posters in shopping malls and airports. Many are the victims of broken marriages and have become the pawns in their parents' struggles with each other. But others are just victims. They disappear without warning from public places — airports, playgrounds and schoolyards. They're sometimes found and returned with the fresh wounds of molestation and assault, scars that never completely heal. Sometimes they're unearthed in shallow graves. Perhaps even worse, sometimes they disappear from the face of the earth, never to be seen or heard from again. Are they dead or alive? There are no explanations, no good-byes. How do you grieve when there's no body?

"I'll report it to the information desk, Don." The clerk listened intently to my story. Even before I had finished, her fingers were dialling a familiar number. "I'll get you the police. They should be informed at once."

Time was of the essence. If Matthew had been kidnapped, every minute was vital. Once a car left the airport he could disappear forever into the sprawling metropolis of Honolulu. I felt sick. Don's eyes were wild with fear. The lady handed the phone over to me.

"Yes, ma'am, you have a problem?" The voice was authoritative. I imagined him poised over a form headed "Missing Persons."

"Child's name?"

"Matthew James Ekroth."

"Age?"

"Five years, three months."

"Colour of hair?"

"Brown."

"Colour of eyes?"

"Blue."

This is a bad dream, I thought. It can't be real. This was the stuff of TV drama. It had no place in our ordinary lives. I was shaking uncontrollably.

"How long has he been missing?"

And then, from the corner of my eye, I saw him. He was being led out of the dining area by the clerk from the information desk. She had joined the search for him, too, and somehow had found him playing with the cigarette machines. Content in a world of his own, he was oblivious to the energy being expended on his behalf.

"Where have you been?" Don's voice was loud and angry, relieved beyond words. "We've looked everywhere for you. Why did you go away? Mom's on the phone to the police about you right now. And where on earth were you?'' He might well ask. Don had searched the dining area three times without success.

"Someone could have taken you. They could have hurt you or killed you. We might have lost you forever.'' Curious travellers paused to stare. Matthew, suddenly grasping the severity of the situation, started to cry.

"How long has he been missing, ma'am?'' the policeman repeated.

Relief seeped through every cell of my body. Suddenly exhausted, I explained that Matthew had been found. The Missing Persons form for Matthew James Ekroth was crumpled up and discarded. Don delivered an immediate, essential, and significant spanking, then, grabbing our hand luggage, we raced to the gate to catch our flight back to Vancouver.

"The plane's about to leave,'' an attractive flight attendant told us. She spoke into her hand radio. "They're here,'' was all she said. There was a garbled reply. "They're waiting. You'll have to rush.'' The enormous door re-opened and we fell into the aircraft. Hundreds of eyes zeroed in, and followed our progress to the four empty seats.

The Hawaiian Islands were still in sight as we downed our second stiff drink. "I really thought we'd lost him,'' I whispered to Don. "I couldn't bear it, could you?''

Chapter Three

I'm leaving on a jet plane,
Don't know when I'll be back again,
Oh babe, I hate to go

Matthew is sitting on the couch in the family room, playing his favourite John Denver tape. Tears run down his face. I've seen this before, but feel obliged to ask anyway.

"Why are you crying, guy?"

"I dunno. It just makes me cry."

"Well, sometimes there's a thin line between beauty and sadness," I tell him, leaving him to his solitude.

It's spring, 1985. Elizabeth, now seven, is in grade one and Matthew's in kindergarten. His social skills are improving steadily, and each morning, he literally jumps out of the car to race across the school field in anticipation of another exciting day.

Both Elizabeth and Matthew are enroled in Scottish Highland dancing classes. Their teacher, Marilyn Merry, injects large measures of humour and love into her lessons, and both children enjoy them immensely. Boys are a rare commodity in Highland dancing, and as such, enjoy a special status. Matthew positively glows with all the attention.

Elizabeth is in Brownies, Matthew in Beavers. Life is full and rich and bright with promise. There are no dark clouds on our horizon. Emotionally, physically and financially, we feel like the chosen people.

After an eight-year absence, I return to nursing. The only feasible option is casual on-call — far from ideal, but it's a foot in the door. Delta Hospital is small and friendly. I'm glad to be back, but I have trouble with the new terminology. Since when did a patient become a "client?" And "modules," "conceptual frameworks," "nursing processes?" Spare me. Just show me the patient, the bedpans, the drug cupboard and let me get on with my work. Often the real medicine is our time: time to listen, to understand, to care.

Don is on a natural high that all fishermen recognize and share. He's preparing for the salmon season, which, for gillnetters, starts in June. This year's runs are predicted to be the best in years. He has been planning the season since January, and is well into the tasks of mending nets, making annual repairs, checking out electronics and a myriad of minor preparations.

Matthew finishes school at lunchtime, so each afternoon we have some time together. Frequently one of his little friends — Robert, Gregory or Austin — will come and play, but often it's just the two of us. We love Diefenbaker Park, a large rolling hollow with a generous artificial pond in the middle. A waterfall tumbles down from a hilly ridge and assembles at the bottom to become a stream, which then meanders into the pond. Frogs and tadpoles know it as home; little boys know it as paradise. Further along the ridge, trees and shrubs conspire to conceal lurking monsters. Our friend Winnie the Pooh could be anywhere. We must find and save him. The story ends happily, so we race down the hill for a few minutes' play on the slide and monkey bars. The little wooden bridge is perfect for a game of Three Billy Goats Gruff. I usually play the part of the troll.

"Who's that clip-clopping over my bridge?" (It's more fun than being a goat!) It's three o'clock, time to pick Elizabeth up from school.

"I'm so glad we have this time together," I tell him. He smiles, but his look reminds me that there is a time and place to get mushy with a mother and this isn't one of them.

At bedtime, having finished his prayers, he becomes thoughtful and serious. His large eyes are brimming with unspilt tears. "Mommy, where do we go when we die?"

I'm totally unprepared. What brought this on?

"We go to heaven when we die, Matthew. Jesus has promised that if we love Him, we can live with Him forever."

"But will we be together?" He is sobbing now.

"Yes, I believe we will, though I don't know for sure. But the one thing I do know is that it will be all right. There will be no pain, no illness, no sadness; we'll just be happy and peaceful." Matthew has crawled from under his covers and is curled up on my lap. We are rocking back and forth together. It's as natural to kiss his soft brown hair as it is to breathe in and out.

"But will we look the same, Mommy?"

"I don't know, Matthew. There are lots of questions to which we don't know the answers. When we die, the spirit leaves the body. The spirit is the part that makes you Matthew, and me the person I am, and Dad and Elizabeth into the people that they are. It's actually separate from the body. When our bodies don't work properly anymore — and that's usually when we're old — they die and change, but our spirits live on and go to heaven."

"But how will I know you? And how will you know me?"

"I don't know, son. I just know that we don't need to worry about it. God takes care of it all."

"But I don't understand, and it's scary."

"It's very hard to understand, guy. Even adults don't fully understand. You don't remember being a little baby, do you? You were curled up inside my tummy. You had eyes, ears, a nose, a mouth, hands and feet, and all your other parts. If you had been able to think about it at the time, you would probably have asked, 'Why am I like this? I live in a dark, warm, wet home, and don't need this body. I don't understand!' And then, of course, what happened?''

"I got born."

"That's right. You came out into the world. And the first parts you needed were your lungs. You needed to breathe. And then you needed your mouth. You were hungry and had to drink some milk. And you used your eyes to see, and your ears to hear. In fact, there was indeed a purpose for every part of your body. At the time you couldn't have imagined what the world was like, could you? And I believe it's the same when we die. At this stage it's hard to imagine what heaven is going to be like. And it's very hard to imagine what we will be like if we leave our earthly body behind. But even though we don't fully understand, we have God's promise that we will be well taken care of.''

"But do we have to stay in heaven?" I think Matthew pictured heaven as being a town like Tsawwassen. I'm not sure I was successful at conveying my own concept of a boundless expanse.

"But do dogs go to heaven?"

I begin to feel I'm on more familiar territory.

"I don't know, guy. I just know that everything is going to be all right.''

He gives me a big hug and kiss and I snuggle him beneath the covers.

This conversation becomes an obsession, repeated in varying forms over the next few weeks. I couldn't know then how grateful I would be in the months ahead for these opportunities to share with him while we were both on safe ground.

It's finally June. The days are warm and the evenings light; the sounds of lawnmowers awaken memories of summers past. Gardens have burst into colour, and trees are proudly dressed in various shades of green. There is a general feeling of winding down and of lazy days ahead.

I had been seeing Matthew's kindergarten teacher each Friday to briefly discuss progress, or the lack thereof, in the behaviour department, and now it's report card time. I have promised that if it's good, we'll go and pick out a present from the toy shop. His anxious face is close to mine.

"Read it, Mom, read it."

I glance through the typed lines. Somehow everything has come together.

Matthew has been one of my little sunshines for the past two months.

He is very keen, and makes full use of all the French vocabulary he has learned.

He always participates in oral conversations and he has made excellent progress in maintaining good behaviour. He is extremely affectionate and I have thoroughly enjoyed him.

Good luck in grade one, Matthew!

"Yippee, Mom! There's a new Transformer I want. Optimus Prime is awesome. Let's go." I have to explain to him that thirty-five dollars was not the amount I had in mind for the occasion. We compromise, I hug him and tell him he should feel very proud. At last, we are well on our way.

"Granny Petal" is here from England to spend five weeks with us, and the children are in heaven. Here's someone who seems to live only to dispense stories, hugs and gum. My mother's conversion to the joys of gum is fascinating to me, since as children we were never allowed it. Never!

Don is away salmon fishing in Barkley Sound. He comes home every two or three weeks, but we don't plan around him, as the salmon runs — and consequently his schedule — are unpredictable. We do our thing, and when he's home, he slides into our activities and it's a bonus.

There's excited talk of waterslides, trips to the beach, and vacation bible school. I have enroled both children in swimming lessons. Now if Matthew can only shake this cough, the summer will be perfect.

The Highland dance competition is on the first Saturday of the holiday, but it turns out that only Elizabeth and I go. Matthew's cough is troublesome.

He's disappointed to miss the competition, but pale and tired, he gives in easily to the prospect of watching cartoons with Granny Petal. As I kiss the top of his head, I notice that he has again abandoned his favourite chair. He's sitting on the living room floor leaning forward on the footstool — the first of many clues that I fail to recognize as important.

"Mommy, do my hair, please."

Elizabeth is wearing a lovely purple and white plaid kilt with a matching purple jacket. I groan inwardly. Her blond hair just reaches her shoulders. She'll lose marks if I leave it loose, but it's too short to put up easily. There's no choice. A dozen bobby pins, a hair net and half a can of hair spray later, we're finally ready to leave.

We arrive at the competition at the same time as Marilyn Merry, the children's dance teacher. I tell her Matthew is not well enough to dance today. She's not surprised.

"Yes, I noticed that he seemed to be short of breath and wheezing in his lesson this week. Poor Matthew! Good luck, Beth. Now don't forget to point your toes."

The following Monday, Matthew's cough is no better. He is tired, has no appetite, and is complaining of nausea. Also, he's not arguing with Elizabeth: he must be feeling rotten. I make an appointment for him and we head down to Dr. Martin's office.

Removing the stethoscope from his ears, he calmly says, "I don't hear anything, but we know from past experience how deceptive Matthew's chest can be."

In spite of the implication of his words, I refuse to acknowledge that Matthew's cough could be in any way associated with the frightening X-ray of nearly three years ago. All he needs is a course of antibiotics and he'll be well in no time, I tell myself.

But it's not that easy. Six weeks and three courses of antibiotics later, Matthew still suffers from the harsh, rasping cough.

"He's got bronchitis," I explain to friends. "It's really pulled him down. You don't expect this kind of problem in the summer, do you?"

Many of our marvellous plans have been abandoned and, in compensation, we put extra effort into preparations for Matthew's sixth birthday party.

In the warm sunshine of early afternoon on August 20, the young guests arrive. Matthew has an awful cough, but after all the antibiotics, I'm sure he's not infectious.

"Yes, he has lost weight, hasn't he?" I tell half a dozen mothers. "He doesn't feel like eating anything. If it weren't for Chicken McNuggets, I don't know where we'd be."

I had volunteered to serve as nurse for one day of the Alliance Church vacation bible school, and the following morning, we rise early and get ready. Matthew is coming along. He's officially too young for camp yet, but I know he'll enjoy the other kids and, in spite of his lethargy, some of the quieter activities.

Sure enough, within a few minutes he's best buddies with an older boy. They blend into the sea of young faces and I turn my attention to medical duties.

"You probably won't have much to do," Darlene, one of the organizers, tells me as I check through the first-aid box. "There's usually just the odd scratch or two."

After a few hours and an avalanche of minor ailments, I'm exhausted! As the kids attack their lunch, I have my first chance to sit down and think about getting through the rest of the day.

Lunch done, the youngsters board the camp bus for the two-mile trip to the local pool. Matthew knows that he can't swim because of his cough, but he badly wants to ride on the bus with his new friend.

But the bus is full. "Next year, son," I give him a consoling hug. "You'll be old enough next year."

Campfire is the favourite time of day. Sleepy, grubby bodies lean against each other as the light from the flames dances from face to face.

A general feeling of contentment and camaraderie settles over the gathering. I, too, am pleasantly tired from the day's activities. As the group leader weaves the magic of a campfire story, my eyes drift lazily from child to child, each one held in rapt attention in the half-light. All eyes are on the group leader, all imaginations carried away on the fire's sparks.

For no conscious reason, my eyes come to rest on one little boy. Sitting close to a friend, totally immersed in the story, his gaunt frame stands out in sharp relief against the tanned, robust bodies of the other boys. His large, serious eyes are sunk deep into the shadows of his face. He's leaning forward in an unusual position, as if by necessity. He's obviously very ill. Anyone can see that.

Matthew. My peaceful world shatters like glass. The child is Matthew! When did this happen? Why haven't I noticed before? Shocked, I re-examine the once-familiar face.

I know he hasn't been eating much, but could he really have lost this much weight? I know his chest has been congested, but how could I not have seen his obvious difficulty in just breathing?

I become vaguely aware that the story is now finished. The closing prayer includes a blessing for tomorrow's camp activities. I resolve that my tomorrow will be spent in addressing the problems that have become so painfully evident tonight.

After lunch, I take a chair from the kitchen and sit on the back patio in the sunshine. It's the last day of vacation bible school and Elizabeth is there, involved in preparations for tonight's parents' concert. Don is down at the river preparing his boat for the opening of the salmon season. The sockeye bound for the Fraser River are expected in record numbers this year, so there is much excitement. Matthew is staging a space battle, darting indoors and out.

Yesterday I had taken him to Dr. Martin, and expressed my concerns about the cough that had persisted through the rounds of antibiotics. I hear Matthew's voice now, alternately talking and making sound effects, playing out the roles of first the good guys and then the bad. Maybe I was overreacting. Dr. Martin had ordered X-rays — just routine, but best to be on the safe side, he reassured me. I thumb through my magazine, savouring the moment, and turn my mind to the change of routine school will soon bring. I find myself daydreaming.

Somewhere in the distance a phone rings. A minute later, Matthew trails out to the patio. "Mommy, Dr. Martin's on the phone."

I recall another day, another phone call. Long-forgotten memories resurface and I push them back.

"Hello, Dr. Martin."

"Hello, Mrs. Ekroth. Well, I've looked at Matthew's X-rays with the radiologist. I'm afraid it appears that there are some serious problems." I don't hear it all. ". . . fluid in the lungs . . .liver enlarged. . . congestive heart failure. . . Dr. Mirhady's office right away. . . Children's Hospital."

I am frozen, rooted to the spot. I dare not move in case I fall. Fear stabs savagely and without mercy. I concentrate on finding a calm voice, on maintaining some control. What comes out is distant, choked, breathless.

"Do we know what is causing this, Dr. Martin?"

"No, I'm afraid we don't." He repeats the need to take Matthew to Dr. Mirhady immediately. "Can you do that?" he adds gently.

The same distant voice replies, "Yes. Goodbye. Thank you, Dr. Martin."

For what seems like a long time, I stand motionless; external functions shut down as I try to absorb what I have just heard. I feel numbed and dull, yet aware of some unfamiliar inner workings creaking into action to shore me up against this unbearable assault. I want to shout, to scream, to throw and break something, to vehemently protest the unfairness of life, to pull it back into balance. Instead, I weep tears of devastation and phone Don's Mom.

Matthew packs a small overnight bag with the necessities of life — Doggy and blankie, two Transformers, some colouring books and crayons. I add his pyjamas, toothbrush and toothpaste.

I am hiding behind extra make-up and a pair of sunglasses. Thankfully, I have regained some control. Matthew is nonchalant. He expresses no feelings and asks no questions. I have never loved him more.

The same friendly receptionist. The same examination room. The same circus animals on the wallpaper. The same painstaking, meticulous examination by Dr. Mirhady. Today, he's very quiet.

"Breathe in, Matthew." He scans the little boy's chest with his stethoscope, listening intently. He doesn't smile.

Finally, Matthew disappears into the waiting room to play, and Dr. Mirhady brings out a folder bearing the incriminating X-ray.

"Have you seen this?" he asks.

"No." I'm not sure I want to. He holds it up to the light and I stare in horrified fascination. In my twelve years as a nurse, I've seen many chest X-rays, but never one that even vaguely resembled this. Both lungs exhibit gross, dark patterning throughout. The pleural cavity — the space between the lungs and the chest cavity — also shows abnormal dark shadows. The heart, liver and spleen are all enlarged.

"It appears that the problem has become much worse. We will have to admit our friend Matthew to Children's Hospital and find out what is causing his illness."

I nod miserably, hoping against hope that Dr. Mirhady can supply some explanation, some diagnosis. His silence confirms my worst fears. Again I hear the unfamiliar voice, feel the dry burn of fear. "Do you have any ideas as to what could be causing this, Dr. Mirhady?"

He pauses momentarily, choosing his words with care. "We cannot know until we have done some tests. But the first thing I want to rule out is Hodgkin's disease." Hodgkin's disease, I scream inwardly. Cancer of the lymph system. Matthew's only six. Why him? Why us? No, it isn't possible.

Dr. Mirhady has more bad news. It is Friday and the hospital diagnostic facilities are only open for emergencies. We have to return home. Matthew will be admitted on Monday. I can hardly stand the thought. How on earth are we going to get through two days at home knowing what we do? I desperately want him to start the tests and subsequent treatments now, not in two days' time. Hodgkin's disease has to be ruled out as soon as possible. Doesn't he know we can't wait two days?

We join the stream of traffic leaving the city at rush hour. It is especially heavy tonight, as people head for the ferries to Vancouver Island or the Gulf Islands. Workers released from their offices to the warm August afternoon are impatient for the freedom of the weekend — maybe a last chance to use the pool and barbecue before autumn puts in an appearance. Summer's nearly over, but we can catch the last act if we hurry.

Hurry up and wait. We crawl along, brake lights constantly flashing. The little boy sitting by my side is pale and quiet. Resigned. We have no need to talk. He has chosen our favourite tape, and Roger Whittaker sings "The Balladeer." Tears course down my face. If Matthew notices, he doesn't comment. Already we are learning how to protect each other.

The trip home seems to last forever. I'm strangely aware that we have just embarked on a different kind of journey, the route and destination of which are frighteningly uncertain.

Don arrives home from the river. His parents have tracked him down to advise him of this new threat to his son. His eyes are fearful, searching. We escape to the privacy of our bedroom, and I tell him all I know. I watch in agony as he reels from the blow. Broken hopes, shattered dreams, unthinkable possibilities for the future. Already our grief has begun.

Saturday is spent in a scurry of activity preparing for the days ahead. Delta Hospital is alerted that I won't be free for on-call duty for a while. Family in England and close friends are phoned, and share our pain. There is shopping to be done — new pyjamas and dressing gown for Matthew, new sitting-in-hospital clothes for me.

The Fraser River fishery is scheduled to open at eight o'clock Sunday morning. On the spur of the moment, we decide to make it a family outing, the first of many treasured times together over the next year. We plan to leave home on Saturday evening and sleep on the boat overnight. The children are both excited at the prospect of such an adventure.

The Fraser River is renowned as the greatest salmon river in the world. Gillnetters converge in large numbers to intercept the millions of salmon migrating toward their spawning grounds, almost five hundred miles upstream. It's an exciting time to be involved in the fishing industry — the peak of the run, good prices and good weather all combine to make the fishing openings lucrative. It's during this short time that the majority of our year's income will be made.

The children snuggle into their bunks and are asleep in minutes. Don and I lie awake for a long time, listening to the sounds of the river and grappling with our fears and sadness. Don sleeps fitfully and is up early checking everything one more time. The immense river shimmers in the early morning sunshine. The thin haze hovering above the surface won't last long on a glorious day like this.

Don feigns an air of calm as he finishes breakfast. He has run the *Sunburst* downriver to a fishing spot he knows well. The gillnetters are lined up on both sides of the river. Each fisherman jealously guards his area, and tempers quickly flare if a latecomer should attempt to trespass.

Conversations over the radio are short.

"You there, Al? Got the right time?"

"Yep, I make her six minutes to go. I think I can see where you are, Joe. Just watch out for that boom behind you. That corner can be a real bugger when it's running this hard."

The radio telephone is noticeably silent as the final minute to countdown approaches. Fishermen, now in the stern, are alert and ready for business. Elizabeth and Matthew, sporting orange life-jackets, stand on the hatch close to Don, and survey the scene around them.

"Can I fish when I'm older, Dad?" Matthew asks.

"We'll see," Don replies, but dares not meet his son's eyes.

The radio telephone crackles again.

"Attention, all fishermen. This is the Fisheries patrol vessel Heron Rock . . ." The remainder of the Fisheries officer's message is drowned out by the roar of engines. The gillnetters manoeuvre across the water, each streaming 1,200 feet of net in their wake. This first set is crucial. It may be the only good catch of the opening. Once the nets are out, the tension is strangely diffused and the fun part begins.

"Come on, fishy, fishy, fishy," encourages Elizabeth.

"There's one," Matthew yells. The corkline bounces as a shimmering salmon twists and struggles in the web directly beneath. Here and there the corkline dances in the sunlight, announcing the arrival of scores more of his comrades. How amazing! In spite of everything, life can still be good.

The tide is running at four to five knots as the net drifts downstream toward the massive expanse of the Port Mann Bridge. Don needs all the knowledge and experience of his twenty-six years in fishing to protect his net and its catch. Log booms lining the river, and their accompanying snags of errant logs and driftwood on the riverbed, can reduce a net to ruins in a matter of seconds. He guards and tends it, controlling its passage and protecting it from harm.

"Mom, I feel sick and dizzy." Matt is sitting on the hatch. His eyes are dull, his lips blue-tinged, his breathing laboured. I am sadly reminded that where he's concerned, we have lost control and the ability to protect.

Later in the day, Don radio-telephones Children's Hospital to confirm that Matthew has a bed for tomorrow. He drops the two of us off near the car and we drive back home for the night. Elizabeth stays on board. She has become the "official fish counter." That night at home, I snuggle Matthew into bed and wait to hear his prayers. Nothing and no one is forgotten — the poor, the sick, the sad, the lonely, the animals. The list of needy causes is endless. Finally, he comes to the subject that permeates my every waking thought: "and please help me get better, and please help me not be nervous in the hospital."

I jump on that, the perfect opening to discuss such fears as operations, needles and IVs.

"And what are you nervous of in particular, hon?" I ask, confident of being three steps ahead.

"There's just one thing that's bothering me," he confides. He looks away and doodles with his fingers on the shy wallpaper elephants. "I don't want the nurses to see me with my pants off."

"I'll see what we can do, fella," I tell him, and escape before I explode with laughter and relief.

The following morning, Monday, August 26, dawns bright and clear, and promises to be another hot day. Children's Day at the Pacific National Exhibition, I think ruefully. I had planned to take Elizabeth and Matthew; like all kids, they loved the thrills of a fair. It was to have been a last special outing before the back-to-school shopping began.

"What would you like for breakfast, Matthew?" He's watching cartoons on TV in the living room, draped across the footstool to give himself maximum breathing capacity. The position is becoming familiar to me: I've often seen hospital patients with respiratory disease similarly propped up. But they're generally old, I think bitterly.

"Not hungry, Mom," he replies.

"Come on, hon, you have to eat something. It'll help you get better. How about a few Cheerios? As a special treat you can have them in front of the TV." The blackmail works, thank God. He's become so thin I'd resort to anything.

Later in the morning, the doorbell rings. It's Lynn Robertson, the associate minister of our church. She learned about Matthew's problems from a friend at church yesterday and now listens sympathetically, as between sobs, I relate our story. She hugs me tight. "We'll pray for Matthew and your family," she says. I'm glad; I'm far too angry with God to discuss anything with him myself. I leave Lynn in the playroom while I go to answer the phone. Through the kitchen window I can see both Lynn and Matthew clearly. Lynn is standing at the closed patio doors watching Matthew outside in the backyard playing with his bow and suction-tipped arrows. Suddenly he turns and studiously fires one at my benevolent friend. Thunk! It hits the glass patio doors right between her eyes. He throws his head back and roars with laughter. I can't help but smile, and I feel enormous relief that in the midst of chaos, some things remain the same.

"Not hungry, Mom."

It's lunchtime and we're running through our familiar routine.

"You'll have to eat if you want to get better, son." He reluctantly agrees to two slices of cucumber and a small plate of yogurt and honey.

After lunch we check through his hospital bag. He has packed his favourite Transformers, He-Man figures, books and crayons. There is just one more thing left to do. "I want some photos of you, guy," I tell him as casually as possible. We don't know what's ahead, but already I feel a compelling need to collect souvenirs and keepsakes of our son. He poses under the hanging planter at the front door, and I take three pictures, just in case.

Some time later, when the pictures are finally developed, I notice that in all of them, Matthew's arms are stretched up, his hands folded across his red cap. What I took at the time to be a mannerism was a compensatory position that would allow him to breathe a little easier. It will astound me how I could be so blind to such evidence of his condition.

Chapter Four

The Children's Hospital. I had passed it many times, smug in the security of having such a fine facility so close by, yet not imagining any need for it in our lives. It was for other people, the parents with very sick children. Not us.

I try to be bright and casual as we park the car in the lot and head for the main entrance. This, I pretend, is a routine trip, like a visit to the shopping mall. Matthew picks up on the attitude and acts cavalier, striding along in a grown-up way that he's learned by imitating Don. We pause for a minute outside the hospital to study and admire the beautiful tile mosaics — an exercise which serves to reinforce our nonchalance. Matt loves the "magic" doors that open as we approach and is soon immersed in a game in which he assigns himself as "doorman." I realize that I wouldn't normally allow him to monopolize the entrance to a public building, but he's having such a good time — and it's suddenly hard to say no. Fortunately, I'm let off the hook: he's diverted by a baby in the lobby.

"Hello, baby." He strokes the soft, warm down of the infant's head.

A bustling square with seating in the centre and hallways leading off to the various wings, the lobby could be a train station were it not for the wheelchairs and white-smocked health professionals.

A woman with a clipboard writes down Matthew's name. "Please take a seat. We'll call you when it's your turn."

I find an empty place in the crowded seating area, joining other parents with care-etched faces, whispering reassurances to their children as they wait to be admitted. The fear zone. Working on a hunch that the sooner we feel at home, the better, I try to familiarize myself with these new surroundings. Three elevators open and close in front of us, discharging their cargo of doctors, nurses, physiotherapists, dieticians, patients, parents and many others who have come from the inpatient floors above, before scooping up a new group. They are in constant motion. To my left, the hospital cafeteria is visible through glass windows. Most of the tables here are empty now, but soon they'll fill again as the staff begin to take their afternoon coffee breaks. Next door is the gift shop where Matthew gazes, nose pressed against the window, at the assortment of toys, books, and candies inside. The corridor in front of the cafeteria and gift shop leads to the right to the clinic areas, and to the left, to radiology, the operating rooms, laboratories and the intensive care unit, or I.C.U. Behind me, another elevator opens and closes in more leisurely manner; it serves the large underground parking lot. Clerks at the information desk help newcomers make sense of it all. Beyond, at the admitting desk, three clerks feed information into their computers which is, in turn, churned out by the printers behind them.

"Matthew Ekroth," the lady with the clipboard calls.

We sit in front of one of the clerks with the computers. She is neutral as she copies from Dr. Mirhady's admission slip.

Matthew James Ekroth.

Provisional Diagnosis: Lung infiltrate. Malignancy.

She types the information without comment or change of expression. I find myself wondering how she distances herself from the succession of disease and sadness that pauses at her desk each day.

"Matthew will be on 3B. A volunteer will be along to take you up to the floor in a few minutes."

The elevator doors open onto 3B and the end of innocence. Shuffling slowly toward us is a very pale girl pushing an IV pole ahead of her. I guess her to be seven or eight years old.

"Mom," Matthew whispers, "where's her hair?" He stares at the child. The reality hits me broadside; I have no idea what Matthew is thinking. This is oncology — the cancer ward. It shouldn't shock me like this! I know they want to test for Hodgkin's disease, but please God, I'm not ready for this!

We are shown to a four-bed room. There is one other little boy in the opposite bed and we soon learn his name is Mike. There is nothing to do but make the best of the situation.

"Oh, isn't this a nice, bright room, Matt," I twitter. "Look, you can even see the mountains from here. This is your bed, right by the door. And look, you have your own locker for your clothes and another for your toys, so you can play with them any time you want. Oh, and look, Matt, you're right beside the sink and there's a lovely little bathroom in here. Come and see. Look, Matt, there's a TV. You'll be able to watch 'He-Man' and 'Transformers.'" Mike nods agreement.

"Well, aren't you lucky? I think I'll see if there's an extra bed for me." I babble on as we busy ourselves with unpacking and getting settled. My mind races ahead, plotting to find a private place to cry.

A pretty, smiling nurse takes Matthew to be weighed and measured for height. They are friends by the time they reach the door. I wander out into the hall to orient myself to our new surroundings. My attention is drawn to the bulletin board where a pamphlet, showing a woman crying on a man's shoulder, stares back at me. Other notices tell of support groups for the parents of terminally ill children and shops where wigs may be bought locally.

"Hello, you must be Matthew's mom. I'm Jan Mitchell, the social worker."

I turn around to meet a petite young woman. Our first eye contact tells me that she is not fooled by my facade. The sorrow, so carefully corralled, explodes in a flood of tears.

"We can talk in my office," she says, gently leading me down the corridor.

At last, a refuge. Falling into her easy chair, I bury my face in a wad of tissues and sob. Jan waits. She waits for a long time.

Eventually I splutter through my misery. "I can't stop crying. How can I talk to the doctors? How can I be strong for Matthew? I just can't stop crying." Jan nods sympathetically.

"This stage is one of the most difficult for any parent," she reassures me. "You suspect that Matthew is seriously ill, but don't know what's wrong yet, or what you have to deal with. There's something else too. It's important for you to know early on that marriages can suffer greatly under the stress of dealing with a very sick child. Contrary to popular belief, this situation doesn't often draw a couple closer together. In fact, it often puts an enormous strain on the relationship. I'm not trying to add to your trouble, but I like parents to understand the problems right from the beginning."

Jan pauses while I blow my nose loudly. My eyes are burning, my face is hot. I know I must look awful.

"I'd like to make a suggestion or two that will help you cope through the next few days," she says. "Try not to jump ahead. That can be frightening to say the least, and may be totally irrelevant. Remember, we don't yet know what we have to deal with. Take one day at a time. All you have to deal with is the present. Nothing else."

I soon discover that this is good advice — though even an hour at a time is too long by far on occasion. So I develop a back-up plan. Whenever I feel unable to cope, I focus only on that moment, forbidding myself to see one second beyond. By isolating each activity, my fear of the whole is defused. Not totally, but enough to allow me to function. I can listen to the doctor. I can read Matthew a story. I can hold his hand while blood is taken. . . and on. . . and on. . . Alone, they're manageable. Together they threaten to overwhelm. Yes, "a minute at a time" works well for me.

He-Man and his evil arch-rival Skeletor are in pitched battle when Sheila Pritchard, the head of Matthew's "team," arrives. She is a haematologist, and is English, judging from her accent. She is slim, pretty, and youthful, but dark circles under her eyes attest to the rigours of long hours spent with seriously ill children and their families.

"Hello Matthew, I'm Dr. Pritchard. I just want to listen to your chest and look at your tummy."

Matthew is oblivious to all but his favourite program. "You'll never take me, He-Man," roars Skeletor.

"It'll only take a few minutes, Matthew," she says. He backs over toward the bed, not taking his eyes off his hero.

The short check-up over, he gives his full attention to his program.

"It may be premature of us to have Matthew on this floor," Dr. Pritchard's words are music in my ears. "Once we've done some tests, we'll have a better idea of what we're dealing with. Tomorrow, we'll do some blood work and take some X-rays. Dr. Sandor, our cardiologist, has scheduled an ECG and an echocardiogram of his heart and abdomen as well, to make sure everything is OK. I'll check with you tomorrow." She smiles, nods and moves on.

Her manner carries with it a gentle hint of optimism and I seize it hungrily. In the background, He-Man has triumphed yet again over the evil forces of Skeletor.

Based on this introduction to Dr. Pritchard, I'm heartened by the team of highly-skilled specialists working for Matt. They will soon know what is wrong and, like the good guys, ride in to save the day.

Matthew wanders out to the nurses' station and seeks out Sue, his admitting nurse. "She's decent *and* awesome, Mom," he has already confided to me. High praise indeed. I pass them deep in conversation. Matthew is already at home on the nurses' side of the station. Well, that didn't take him long, I think with amusement. Down the corridor are several more patients' rooms, some with two beds, some with four. Catastrophic illness has no respect for age, and the children range from infancy up to sixteen years.

Most of the younger patients have at least one parent hovering, in varying stages of coping. Their eyes may be red-rimmed and dazed. Some have had more experience at this and know what they are up against. They recite statistics with the authority of a specialist. Long, complex names of drugs roll off their tongues. Normal units of blood work become a second language.

Whatever the odds, the fight is on. Getting through the day requires a strategy. Spontaneity is left behind in another life. Here, words are planned carefully. There are optimistic pep-talks before each battle, cautious interpretations of the doctors' prognosis afterward. There's a lot of hugging, hand-holding and loving on this floor. It's important to say the things we need to say to our precious children. We want no legacy of guilt or regret. We have to make each day count — we suspect that they may already be numbered.

Through it all, we cling to our one ally, hope. As one hope fades, another rises to stand in its place. We know the danger of hoping too much, yet we can't put one foot in front of the other without having some hope, no matter how small. We hope for a miracle, or just for a peaceful ending. Without hope we would despair.

At the far end of the corridor, the door opens out onto the flat roof of the hospital. Two children play in the sandbox in the late-afternoon sunshine while their mothers sit close by, deep in quiet conversation, bonded by their mutual torment. Their faces are pale with exhaustion and strain.

I wander over to a large swinging seat near the perimeter of the garden area and gratefully collapse onto it. There is no one else around. This will be the place — I have found my perfect spot to cry. From here I can look down on the front of the hospital complex. I can see the rush-hour traffic building up along Oak Street, as weary commuters head for home: a normal end to a normal day. How I wish we were still a part of that world. I will never take it for granted again.

When I return to Matthew's room, the evening medications have been given. Friends and relatives have left for the night. Weary mothers are preparing makeshift beds by their sleeping children. I have come prepared to do the same, but Matthew seems content and settled, and I suspect that to stay would be more for my benefit than for his.

The air is warm, even at this hour. I point the car towards home, thankful for the opportunity to give vent to my overwhelming sadness.

The morning sun streaming through the window promises another beautiful day. We would normally be heading for the waterslides, or a picnic in Stanley Park, I think ruefully. The phone rings by my ear.

"Hi Mom." It's Matthew.

"Hello, hon, how are you this morning?"

"Good."

"Are you phoning from the nurses' station?"

"No. I'm using the Snoopy phone. We can use it any time we want. Can I speak to Dad?"

"No, I'm afraid you can't. He's still away fishing on the river. And Beth is still over at Auntie Lonnie's."

"Mike and I have been watching cartoons. Early, really early."

"Well, that's OK. If you have to be in hospital, you might as well enjoy yourselves. I'm being a morning slug, as usual. I'm just getting up now. I'll be in to see you shortly."

A pause, and then, with lowered voice, Matthew gets down to the real business.

"Guess what, Mom."

"What, dear?"

"The nurse came, and asked me to do a you-know-what in a you-know-what."

This is obviously serious stuff.

"Well, that's all right, dear. The nurse just tests it. Everyone has to have that done."

"And Mom. . ."

"Yes, dear?" This is the big one.

"I had some blood taken this morning. I didn't like it much."

"No that's not much fun. But you can cope with that, can't you?"

"She gave me a band-aid with a happy face."

"Well, just try to enjoy the good parts, and we'll cope with the rest together. OK?"

"OK, Mom. Bye now."

"Bye, love. See you soon."

The next hour is a panic. The phone rings constantly — friends and family inquiring, supporting, encouraging. Joy arrives at the door with warm muffins. Don calls from the river. He'll be finished fishing later today and will come to the hospital tonight. The fishing's incredibly good. We should be ecstatic, but it's somehow no longer important.

A new doctor is examining Matthew when I arrive on 3B. Slipping into his curtained cubicle, I watch her closely for hints of revelation. But nothing. Matthew responds to her friendly small-talk, happy to cooperate. She finally pulls the stethoscope free from her ears and folds it quickly, thrusting it into the large pocket of her white hospital coat. She reaches for Matthew's pyjamas top — emblazoned with Transformers — and, seeing he wants no help, turns her attention to me.

"Dr. Fiorillo," she says by way of introduction, extending a hand across Matt's bed. "I work with Dr. Sandor in Cardiology. We're planning an ECG and echocardiogram for Matthew. I was just explaining to him that neither of these tests will hurt. Right, Matthew?" She winks conspiratorially at her young patient. "No needles, remember?" She turns from the bed, tactfully lowering her voice.

"They will tell us much about the state of Matthew's heart," she says. "He'll be going down as soon as possible."

It suddenly occurs to me that there is a small — unlikely yes, but perhaps just the smallest — chance that his heart is the cause of all his problems. Hearts are often repairable. Please, God, please let it be his heart!

Several times during the day I hear myself talking to different friends on the phone. "We're hoping that maybe the valves in his heart aren't working properly. . ." "Wouldn't it be wonderful if there's something wrong with his heart. . ." "Maybe an obstruction in the blood vessels between the heart and lungs. Oh, I do hope so. . ." I must sound like a babbling idiot. Do my friends think I'm deranged? No one hints as much.

Matt is picking at his supper when Dr. Sandor, the cardiologist, arrives on the floor. He is a tall, handsome man with dark hair and eyes to match. In a quiet, sympathetic manner, he tells me that, apart from enlargement of Matthew's heart, there is nothing abnormal. They have tried to find something wrong, but failed. He doesn't apologize in so many words, but I sense he is deeply disappointed too.

"Thank you, Dr. Sandor," I say.

He leaves, taking all hope with him, and I retreat hastily to my outdoor refuge. Far below, another evening rush hour is underway.

Now what? The list of ruled-out diagnoses gets longer, but we seem no closer to the truth. What perverse force is at work, conspiring to make any diagnosis, even the worst possible one, a relief from this tormenting uncertainty?

Some time later, sunglasses securely in place, I return to Matthew's room. He is nibbling on a banana while he watches TV. He's in an irritable mood and merely grunts at my greeting, flinching at the customary kiss on his head.

"Strange," I think, "but then again, maybe not. I'd be pretty grumpy myself, cooped up in hospital on a sunny August day, being poked and prodded — and uncertain of the next move." It was probably just as well that I couldn't see ahead — for, as it turned out, this was merely a taste of what was yet to come.

A new patient has joined Matthew and Mike. In the bed next to Matt's is a beautiful child with dark wispy curls and large serious eyes. Judging from the conversation as the chemotherapy nurse adjusts his IV, the little boy is an old hand at this. A man and an older boy stand by the bed, patting, comforting. After the nurse leaves, we introduce ourselves.

Bradley is four and has had leukemia for a year. They live in Kamloops, three hundred miles from Vancouver. Each time he needs treatment, one parent brings him down while the other stays home and works. There is a mortgage to be paid; life must go on. Whenever Bradley is in Children's Hospital, the family stays at the Easter Seal House, a few minutes' walk away. Yes, it is difficult. And, yes, it is disruptive, but there is no choice. And with each treatment comes new hope.

I am beginning to understand the infinite lengths to which we will go to sustain hope.

Our friend Geraldine arrives with Robert and Andrea. The children are awkward and shy at first, until Matthew assumes his role as tour director and runs through his blood pressure cuff and "magic" bed routine. His guests are suitably impressed. Bradley starts crying loudly; his IV is not working and needs to be restarted. We escape to the fresh evening air on the deck. Bradley's brother has a soccer ball with him and the three boys soon have a game underway. Geraldine and I sink onto a nearby bench.

"Robert is very concerned that the doctors find out what is wrong with Matthew," she tells me. "He says he doesn't want him being put to sleep like his rabbit was." It feels good to laugh, even if it is a little close to the mark.

Geraldine is a trained social worker with experience in working with families in situations such as ours. I'm reluctant to talk at first, fearing that I may start crying again and be unable to stop. I gingerly experiment with a few sentences and thankfully find myself in control. The words tumble out in rapid succession, one feeling trampled by another. There is scarcely time to draw a breath. All that I needed was someone to listen, and no one listens better than Geraldine. Thank God for good friends.

Don and Elizabeth arrive on the scene. While Elizabeth and Matthew argue over who will ride in the wheelchair, I update Don with a medical report. The next step is a big one. Matthew is going to O.R. tomorrow. The surgeon, Dr. Jacques Le Blanc, is planning to do a lung biopsy and drain the surplus fluid from his pericardium. The lung biopsy will give us a diagnosis. At last, we will have some answers.

Darkness falls on another day. We kiss our young man goodnight and head home again. There's a casserole waiting for us on the doorstep, and flowers in the mailbox. The telephone rings as we open the door, and we spend the next hour being bolstered by friends.

But the night is far too short. Don's alarm goes off before dawn, and he and Elizabeth leave for the river. It has been a difficult decision for him to make. His natural inclination is to be at the hospital, to be close to Matthew, to be a support to me. Matthew will be unconscious for most of the day, oblivious to his whereabouts and to those who hover anxiously nearby. The other significant fact is money. Most of our annual income is earned at this time of year. The salmon are here now. They follow their own timetable, inflexible to the whims and problems of humans.

"Go, hon," I tell him. "Let's try to keep things as normal as possible. There's no point you just hanging around the hospital all day."

I arrive at 3B at eight o'clock. Mike and Bradley are picking at food on their breakfast trays. Matthew is colouring in his He-Man book. There is a large "Nothing By Mouth" sign above his bed. He is cool, distant, and waiting for an explanation. I tell him as gently as I am able, choosing my words carefully, trying to portray the operation as a means to being well again. His eyes are brimming with tears, but he refuses to share his anger and fear. He suddenly jumps off the bed and takes shelter in the bathroom. On emerging, he is sullen and resentful. He avoids eye contact, working hard to widen the gap between us.

"Hello, Mrs. Ekroth? And Matthew? I'm Dr. Le Blanc. I will be doing Matthew's surgery today." Dr. Le Blanc, in his operating greens, stands next to Matthew's bed, opposite me. I guess him to be around my age. He has a heavy Quebecois French accent. We had already heard much about his exceptional reputation as a surgeon. He starts to outline the day's procedure. Matthew looks as though he's about to explode.

"Mom," he interrupts in his loudest whisper. "Don't talk about me. I don't want people talking about me."

Dr. Le Blanc and I resume our conversation outside Matthew's room.

"We're assuming a new diagnosis," he tells me above the noise of the busy corridor. "We suspect that the patterning on Matthew's lungs is a rare form of hem. . ." The words are lost in the wails of a frightened child. The stretcher passes between us and disappears, finally, through the swinging glass doors.

"Sorry, I missed what you said. Could you repeat that?" I ask. The hall seems hot and airless. I really need to sit down.

"We suspect that the patterning on Matthew's lungs is a rare form of haemangioma," repeats the surgeon. Then, before I can ask, "Haemangioma is an abnormal growth of blood vessels. It's related to the common birthmark, if you like. It is. . ."

"Excuse us. Sorry." A greying woman dressed in the uniform of the hospital Auxiliary manoeuvres her library cart amiably around me. "Sorry, dear," she says again. "Oh, the wheels are stuck. . . there we are now."

"Where were we up to?"

"You were just explaining about haemangiomas." I have a pain in my throat. My voice sounds hoarse and breathless. I move closer to the surgeon, possibly invading his territory. I have to hear his every word.

"Ah yes," he says, backing away a half pace and leaning against the wall. "We have seen haemangiomas in other parts of the body. We have seen them on arms. We have seen them on legs. We have seen them in the abdomen. They can be found anywhere. Even now, there is a baby in I.C.U. with haemangioma on his neck. So it is certainly not unknown. But. . ." The man pauses to choose his words, to shrug his shoulders, to shake his head. ". . .we have never seen it in the lungs before. However," he adds quickly, "let us take one thing at a time. We will not know for sure until we have done the biopsy." I nod my thank-you's as he backs away, not trusting myself to speak.

"I will see you as soon as we are finished," he calls, disappearing toward the elevators. I fight back the rising panic. Don, where are you? Why did I send you fishing when I need you here?

I hear a commotion coming from the bathroom. A nurse retreats, shaking her head and laughing. "Can you believe it? He won't take his underpants off. He's having his bath with his pants on!" She is incredulous. I'm glad for some light relief, but it doesn't last long. Matthew is finally ready for the O.R. The nurse has wrestled his wet underpants away and has dressed him in a hospital gown. He is agitated to the brink of tears.

"I didn't choose this, Mom," he protests emphatically, and I feel my heart breaking. Letting the children make choices was something we'd learned from one of Rudolf Dreikurs's books on child-rearing.

"I didn't choose it either, son. But sometimes we don't have a choice. And we don't have one now." Silently I pray for the O.R. stretcher to arrive immediately, if not sooner — this is all too much for me. In its place our nurse appears at the door.

"I'm afraid they're behind in O.R. It's going to be at least an hour." Matthew is now crying loudly, uncontrollably. I have done all I know. We have talked and prayed and talked some more. I pursue the nurse down the corridor and beg for some sedative for Matt. She promises to phone the O.R. and check with the anaesthetist, although she knows they don't like to give it for this kind of surgery. Within minutes a young man in greens arrives. I don't know who he is, nor do I care. He is working magic with my boy. "Yes, of course you can put your pants on again." "Yes, of course Doggy can come downstairs with you." And "Yes, I'll be with you. I'll be there all the time, Matthew." He disappears, leaving peace and calm in his wake.

The all-important pants are retrieved from the closet, and Doggy from his bedside cupboard. Security restored once more, Matthew leans back against his pillows, tucks Doggy under his arm, and arranges the sheet around them both. His eyes are bright, his face pale. His long dark lashes glisten with the residue of spent tears.

"Here, blow your nose, hon," I tell him, putting a tissue in his hand. "And blow Doggy's too while you're at it. This is hard on all your friends."

The stretcher finally materializes, and transports its small cargo down to the anaesthesia room. As promised, the new friend is waiting. "This is as far as you can come," he tells me kindly.

I kiss Matt's head and say goodbye, and turn before he sees my tears.

Chapter Five

The nurse moves silently around his bed. Checking and charting, monitoring and recording, checking and charting. I sit close by, impotent, redundant, exhausted.

I had been in the I.C.U. waiting room, holding a magazine, when the nurse had come to take me in to see him, warning me, "He has two chest drains, an IV and a blood transfusion. He's on a heart monitor, but don't worry about that — it's just routine after chest surgery. You'll also see that he's very pale. That's mainly because he's loosing a fair amount of blood through the chest tubes. But we're replacing it." She helped me don the mandatory gown and led me through the large I.C.U. to Matthew's bed. Gently, she touched my shoulder, and settled a chair beneath me.

Blip. . . blip. . . blip. . . blip. . . A monitor records the presence of life. The pattern is neat and regular — and infinitely reassuring, for it's the only proof of life in the still, thin boy whose skin is the colour of wax. He lies on his back with his eyes closed. The IV bag contains clear fluid which is fed into a vein in his hand. A second bag holds blood, which drops urgently, first into a plastic chamber, then down toward his splinted arm. Hanging low, at the side of the bed, a plastic container collects and measures the blood that Matthew is losing.

"It's coming through the chest tubes," the nurse points out. "We're hoping the bleeding stops soon." There seem to be dressings everywhere — on his hand, on his arm, and, stained with fresh blood, strapped across his chest. I can smell adhesive and antiseptics, and taste the blood in my mouth.

Now I watch our son dispassionately, as though from a great distance. Like actors on a stage, the people around me act out their parts. The numbness has, of necessity, descended — a filter through which I replay my last conversation with Dr. Le Blanc.

Their suspicions had been correct.

"Diffuse bilateral haemangioma," he had told me. "Small abnormal blood vessels throughout the lung tissue. We have never seen anything quite like it before. It is extremely rare." And then, in answer to my question, "No, it's not malignant. But, in all honesty, it might as well be. We cannot remove it." I listened, but heard no more. I didn't burden him with questions of treatment and prognosis. I already knew the answers.

Don arrives from the river. The white gown is tight around him, and stops a full six inches above his knees. Under different circumstances it would be funny, but no one is laughing now. He touches Matthew's hand and turns, shaking his head. We move away from the bed and find a corner in which to huddle. I pray that the blanket of numbness will quickly enshroud him, too.

Elizabeth is strangely quiet. Matt has had a "satisfactory" post-op night, and Don and I are taking this opportunity to visit with his mom and dad, and, of course, Elizabeth. She doesn't mention her brother's name, and when we volunteer information, she doesn't appear to be interested. Even seven-year-olds develop their own ways of coping.

Poor Elizabeth! There is nothing easy about being a sick child's sibling. It is some weeks later before she tells me how jealous she has been of all the attention Matt is receiving. The constant inquiries, cards, presents, concern — everyone's energy is for Matthew. And as if that wasn't enough, she is bearing her guilt over feeling jealous!

Matthew is under the care of the I.C.U. team as long as he's in the unit, but Sheila Pritchard, as his haematologist, visits him daily. And that is where she finds us on his second post-op day — sitting by his bed, reading cards and unwrapping presents, and adapting as best we can to this new world.

"Hello, Matthew. How are you today?" She has a wonderful way of not "talking down" to children. Matthew tells her exactly how he feels.

"Yes, I know the tubes can be painful, Matthew. Unfortunately we can't remove them while there's so much fluid still draining." She checks the rising Hemovac level, discusses the pain with Ann, who is caring for him today, then turns to Matthew again.

"We can give you a little more medicine for your pain, Matthew. It'll just go in the IV bag so you won't have to have more needles. I'll go and write it up now." Then, turning to us, "perhaps you'd like to come as well so we can talk for a few minutes." Don and I rise as one.

"Well, that was good timing!" Ann, the nurse. "Matt and I have things to do, don't we, Matthew?"

We follow the white coat toward the nurses' station, where Sheila soon locates Matthew's file and checks through the latest reports. Don is chewing the skin around his nails. I am at work detaching myself — taking off my mother's hat and replacing it with the white, starched cap of the nurse. Cool. Professional. Clinical. Much less chance of flipping out.

The station is oddly deserted, with the exception of the ward clerk who is talking on the phone. I find a wall to lean against. Don perches close by on a desk. For a moment, he seems at ease — casual, almost nonchalant.

"Well, he seems to be doing all right at the moment," says Sheila, pulling up a chair. "Dr. Le Blanc talked to you about the diagnosis, didn't he?"

"What kind of prognosis do you think we're looking at?" The unfamiliar voice is mine, the voice of a nurse.

"It's hard to know, Katie," she says. "No one has dealt with this before at Children's. We've really nothing to go on. We found, on the computer, about five or six other instances of children in North America with this disease. The problem is that they were all at different ages and stages of growth, which could make a difference. . ."

"Are the children still alive?" Don. Direct. Deceptively calm. One of his life's hardest questions.

"Well, there's a baby that's still being treated, but. . ." Silence. Just for a moment, but it seems like hours. Sheila grapples for the right words.

"There is, you see, a type of haemangioma that is found mainly in newborns. It's not actually that uncommon. It usually appears as a raised, red mass, and can be anywhere on the body. It can be quite unsightly. New parents get very upset, of course. It does, however, generally disappear within a matter of a few years — and no harm is done." Sheila pulls the white coat around her and crosses her arms, almost protectively.

"And then there's the other kind — the one that just keeps growing. It takes up the space of healthy tissue, and depending on where it is, can be very serious. If it's an arm or a leg that's affected, we've always got the option of amputating, should the growth get out of control. But with lungs. . ." The sentence hangs between us, unfinished. I hear the strange voice again, calm, impersonal. My eyes do not leave Sheila's.

"Would it have made any difference if he'd been diagnosed earlier? He was only two and a half when we first knew his lungs were abnormal. . ."

"Almost certainly not." The reply is fast. No pause, no hesitation. Sheila, I think, has thought this through already.

"You see," she explains, "our options for treatment are very limited. Radiation is a possibility, but the dosage required to affect the blood vessels would likely damage healthy lung tissue. That's the last thing Matthew needs. The other treatment that would have been considered then, as it is now, is steroids. These are drugs that suppress inflammatory reactions, and they might have slowed down the process. I say might. We don't know with this disease. We're doubtful that it would've made any real difference." Don and I glance at each other, sharing this morsel of comfort — one less "if only" to cope with.

"Then I'm glad we didn't know," he says. "We would just have spent those extra years sitting on a time-bomb, unable to do anything. Just waiting. . . How would you ever live with that!''

Three nurses return from their break, relaxed and laughing. Acknowledging our presence, they postpone their joking. They tuck their purses into a cupboard and move quietly away, out into the battleground once more.

"The first thing is to get him over this surgery," Sheila volunteers, correctly anticipating the next question. "As long as there's drainage and the tubes are still in, the major concern is infection. He's already on antibiotics, of course. As for further treatment, there's a team conference tomorrow. Matthew's care will be discussed at length, and we'll get the benefit of everyone's expertise. I'll let you know what comes out of it." Sheila has risen and is returning the chair to its rightful spot.

"I wish we could give you something more definite," she says, "but where Matthew's concerned, we just don't know."

"Thank you," we say. "Thank you very much."

Matthew is sleeping, propped up on pillows. Ann hovers close by, checking fluid levels and filling in a chart. Don resumes his vigil in the armchair, while I rush away to the parents' lounge to cry. The nurse's cap is left behind. I'm Matthew's mom again.

For the next twelve days, we ride an emotional roller coaster. We struggle with our child's pain and his anger. We struggle with our own pain and anger. And we acknowledge the permanent loss of innocence of our young son. We make instant friends in the I.C.U. waiting room, encouraging and being encouraged, comforting and being comforted. We cheer on the doctors. We bargain with God. Our family and friends help to keep us sane: the phone at home rings non-stop, muffins and casseroles arrive daily, prayers are offered in our church and in other local churches, too. We learn of the necessity to live by I.C.U.'s credo, "Take one day at a time." To do otherwise is to be overwhelmed by terrifying possibilities. One day at a time is OK with us. We come home from the hospital each night and sink into exhaustion.

To our relief, we discover ways to regain control, to be able to help. We teach Matthew some simple techniques to deal with pain and fear.

"Blow it away, Matthew. Breathe in slowly, and then imagine that you're blowing away the pain." He is all concentration, and quickly learns how much he can help himself. We all need control.

We also teach him how to escape, if only briefly, from the IVs and the chest tubes.

"Imagine yourself lying on a warm, golden beach. You can be alone or choose to have people with you. Feel the sun on your body. Feel the warm water lapping over your feet. You are relaxed and happy." He is a master of creative visualization. Tension drains from his body. There is a smile on his face.

"You can go to your beach any time you like," I tell him.

It takes little in the way of imagination to realize that the stress of our situation is hazardous to our own health, both mentally and physically. Staying healthy becomes our new goal. Eating well, exercising, sleeping — we can do these for Matt. We're helping indirectly, of course, but that's all right. Every bit helps.

It's the thirteenth day post-op and Matthew is progressing fairly well. The large amount of blood still draining from the two chest tubes is the major concern.

Don has been at the hospital since early morning. I arrive at two o'clock for the afternoon shift, a routine that is working well for us. Don then picks up Elizabeth at three and I stay with Matthew late into the evening.

Gowned and scrubbed, I head for Matt's bed. I.C.U. is strangely quiet. I turn the corner, ready to smile and wave.

I cannot see Matthew. The bed is surrounded by doctors, nurses and a radiologist with a portable machine. Sheila Pritchard is talking in low tones to Dr. Bob Adderley, the I.C.U. doctor. Don and Phyllis, Matt's nurse, have been crying. Everyone stands a little distance from the bed, watching the small, pale child.

I've seen this scenario before as a nurse. It means that everything that can be done has been done. It is now a matter of watching, waiting, hoping, praying.

"Why didn't you phone me, Don?" I am incredulous. I have been folding laundry while Matthew has been fighting for his life.

Dr. Pritchard gives me all the information I need, or can deal with. As feared, Matt has developed a chest infection. The moist condition of his lungs is a perfect medium for the growth of bacteria and the infection is rampant. He started to feel ill late last night and deteriorated during the morning. His pulse is dangerously high, and his blood pressure very low. His condition is critical. He could go either way. He's receiving three different antibiotics intravenously and morphine for pain.

Two hours later, Matthew develops difficulty in breathing. Another X-ray is taken. Fluid is gathering in the pleural space and pressing on his lung tissue. A thoracentesis — removal of the fluid with a large-bore needle — is necessary. Matthew is distressed and frightened, and as the nurses usher us away, we can hear him frantically crying and yelling.

Don and I flee the hospital and find a quiet patch of grass. We weep, together and apart, for a long, long time.

Later, in the kitchen at home — drained, cried out, overwhelmed — we acknowledge this new reality.

"He nearly died today, Don. We almost lost him."

"Yes, I know."

"We have to face that he may die yet."

"Yes, I know."

Don breaks the long silence, slowly weighing every word.

"If he dies, I think we should donate his organs. At least, any organs that can be used. Mind you, I don't expect there'll be a rush on for his lungs."

"Yes, of course," I hear myself agree. "If anything good can come out of this misery, I think we should do it." We hold each other's gaze, gaining new depths of understanding about the person we've been with for the past ten years, hoping maybe that the team dynamic where we take it in turns to buoy each other up will take over now, and one of us will laugh and say, "Hey, you're jumping the gun. Matthew's not going to die."

In the silence that follows, I am reminded of an incident when I was working as an emergency nurse in a hospital in south England. A woman in her late twenties was admitted in a coma, diagnosed as having a brain haemorrhage, and attached to a life-support machine until the full extent of the damage could be assessed. The haemorrhage continued, and a week and three electroencephalograms later, it was determined that she was indeed brain-dead. Permission was obtained to remove her eyes and kidneys, and to donate them for transplantation. The organs were sent to two different London hospitals, and we heard from the surgeon several weeks later that four people had benefited from these gifts. After he'd left, we stood and pondered the miracles of modern medicine.

"Just think, if the family hadn't given permission, those organs would be gone forever," one of the nurses pointed out in her usual blunt manner, "but instead, four people have been given renewed health." It was mind-boggling to us all. Personally, in spite of being a nurse, I had never previously given it more than a cursory thought. It also struck me that in eight months of emergency nursing, this was the first patient I knew of whose organs had been donated. And sadly, many young people with potentially healthy organs either arrived at our doors already dead, or died soon after. The opportunity to retrieve something precious from tragic loss was obviously being missed by many families. One could not fail to see that in organ donation, something good could come from even the worst tragedy. For me, this experience had prompted my filling out a donor card, and shortly after meeting Don, I discovered that he was a potential donor too. But never in our wildest dreams had we considered the involvement of our own children.

The next day is as hopeful as the previous day had been terrifying. An early phone call to I.C.U. tells us that Matthew has had a good night. He's awake and alert and apparently responding to the antibiotics.

We sit at his bedside and hold his hand. He's pale and thin, and the sparkle is gone from his eyes.

"Mom, do you remember saying how much you enjoyed our times together?"

"Yes, Matt. We've had such good times."

"And do you remember saying how much you'd miss it this year when I'm in school all day?" He pauses briefly to catch his breath.

"Yes."

"I'll miss it, too, Mom."

With that his eyes are shut once more. He is fighting for strength. Fighting to live. The wonder and innocence of childhood are gone forever for Matthew. No matter what the outcome, at six years old he has been forced to struggle in life's darkest valley. In his efforts to cope, he is maturing emotionally before our very eyes.

If I have any doubts as to Matthew's awareness of his true condition, they are quickly dispelled. The following evening, Thursday, September 12, turns into a nightmare. He has been on IV morphine for chest pain and needs an extra dose while a chest drain is removed. Within an hour he has a reaction to the extra medication. He hallucinates and becomes dizzy and nauseated. IVs need to be restarted, blood must be taken. All the time his difficulty in breathing increases. Phyllis tries everything she knows, but nothing can stem the steady deterioration. Dr. Bob is called and does all that he can to reverse the situation, and then explains to Matt that we need to do another thoracentesis to drain away more fluid from his lungs. Matt is gasping for breath, but I hear his question distinctly.

"But will I die if I don't get enough air?"

"You'll not die, Matthew," Dr. Bob replies quietly.

"But will I die if I don't get enough air?" Matt repeats. He is panic-stricken. Dr. Bob reassures him as best he can.

"You are getting enough air, Matthew." Within fifteen minutes he has drained off 900 cc's of fluid from the pleural cavity and Matt can breathe easily again. We all breathe easily again.

It is past eleven when I turn the car onto Oak Street for the journey home. The lights are blurred through my tears. I am distraught and angry. For the first time I profoundly realize that while I can be with Matt and help him to the fullest extent of my capabilities, I cannot actually take the experience from him — or spare him from it. I am disgusted with God for the injustice of a little boy's having to cope with something so infinitely horrible. And yet, I can't deny that we are being given many things — an abundance of help and support, the best medical skill and knowledge, and strength we could never have guessed was available to us.

Perhaps the gift for which we are most grateful is Matthew's courage — it is impossible not to admire his fighting spirit. And where does God come into all this? For the life of me I don't understand, but I do know we're not alone.

The crisis passes and Matthew gains a little more strength each day. But they are not easy days. At six years old he is unable to verbalize his feelings or the wide array of difficult and confusing emotions that confront him. Mostly, he is angry. I can't blame him, but it creates a new challenge, as he takes his anger out on me. I try, but fail to understand his motive — he knows how much I love him. Does he blame me for his illness? Does he hold me responsible? I am his mother, yet I failed to protect him. Does he think I should be punished?

"Hi, hon. How are you doing?" He's sitting at a small table in a corner of I.C.U. Don is by his side, knees grazing his chin. Together they're working on a jigsaw puzzle. Don looks up in acknowledgement, but Matthew totally ignores me.

"Say 'hello' to Mom," Don whispers, knowing how much this hurts. A grunt emanates from the bent head.

"So how's it going today?" I ask, as cheerfully as I know how. "Look, there's a piece of the elf's hat."

"Dad and I are doing this!" he snaps.

"Don't be rude, Matthew. Mom was only trying to help."

"Well, we were doing the puzzle, not her." The dulled blue eyes flash with anger. His face is a mask of contempt.

This is a new balancing act to be mastered. At what point do his angry words cross the line between hurt, sick child and rudeness? How wide should the boundaries be set today?

Don's function, at present, is as comforter, friend and playmate. I have drawn the short straw. My role is punching bag. We are a team, each with our own separate duties. Matthew's needs dictate these roles. No, they are not easy days.

Matthew finally comes home on Tuesday, September 24, after a full month in hospital. We are both apprehensive. It's one thing to care for a sick child in a hospital environment; it's another to assume the responsibility at home. He is pale and scrawny, weighing a mere twenty kilos, or forty-four pounds. There is only one way to cope with the uncertainty of our future. Tomorrow doesn't exist. Today is all that matters. It is precious beyond words. Each moment counts.

We tuck our little boy into his bed. He is propped over three pillows to help him breath easier. He closes his eyes tightly and presses his hands together.

"Dear Jesus. Thank you for this day. Thank you that I am getting better. Thank you for our health. . .''

Chapter Six

"Living As If" is the title of a chapter in James Taylor's book *Two Worlds in One*. In it he tells of the life of his son Stephen, who, in spite of an endless regimen of treatments and medication, eventually died of cystic fibrosis at twenty-one years of age. In the wake of the pain and anguish that followed, Stephen's family wondered what the point had been. Why all the effort, struggle and suffering? "Why bother, if failure was inevitable, if it had to end in death anyway?"

Then one day, two months after Stephen's death, James Taylor heard the radio announcement that U.S. forces had invaded Grenada. The danger of Soviet intervention was an ominous possibility. He pondered the situation and wondered what he would do in the event of a nuclear holocaust.

"Nothing, I concluded. I would simply go on living, as best I could, as if whatever I did was worth doing in the time that was left." That sudden realization gave him new insights into why their family's struggle had, in fact, been so important. "Living as if" meant accepting reality, but refusing to be defeated by it, refusing to give up hope even in a hopeless situation. Living as if that hope could be fulfilled.

And so it is with Matthew. We try, and he tries, to live "as if."

On the Sunday following Matthew's discharge, Don's family arrives en masse to see him. "Immediate Family Only" — the rule of I.C.U. — has meant their exclusion from the drama at the hospital. They have phoned, they have prayed, they have cared for Elizabeth. They have thought of nothing else. But they haven't seen Matthew in all this time.

The day is warm and sunny, so I move the chairs outside and arrange them in a circle on the lawn. "They said two o'clock," says Don, "and you know my family — they'll all be on time." At ten to two, the first car pulls up: Grampa and Gramma, closely followed by Lonnie and Bill. Then Don's brother, Lorne, and his wife, Cheryl, with Danielle and Daryl in tow. Lonnie's two sons complete the group: tall, mustached Mike with his wife, Diane, and Mark, now in the police force, with his young fiancee, Lisa. Everyone has taken special pains. They are dressed in their finest. Even Daryl, at nine only happy in jeans and sneakers, has been coerced into a pair of slacks, his blond hair neatly combed. He's on his best behaviour. They hug and kiss us in turn, handing over flowers for me and gifts for the children.

"So where is Matthew?" asks Mom, looking around and lighting her first cigarette. "Tell him Gramma's waiting to see him."

"And Grampa," Pop chimes in, lowering himself into a chair. A large man with a ready smile, Pop has been plagued with asthma for virtually all his life. His breathing is laboured today. Breathing in through his nose, he blows the stale air through his mouth, pursing his lips for better effect. He reaches into a pocket for his Ventolin inhaler — undoubtedly the reason he is still alive today.

Lonnie, Diane, Lorne and Cheryl negotiate for chairs as close as possible to Mom. Our one good ashtray is about to be put to full use.

Leaving Don to distribute drinks, I race inside to see what could be keeping Matt. He's up in his bedroom, changing into the clothes I've chosen for the occasion: a white, collared T-shirt, royal-blue track pants, and a smart grey cardigan enlivened with blue and vivid red stripes. His shirt contrasts with the darkness of his hair, and the blue picks up the colour of his eyes. In spite of his pallid complexion and the way the clothes hang on his thin frame, the picture is a handsome one — a child, appealing and vulnerable.

"Come on, fella. Are you feeling shy?" I ask him, easily sensing the problem. He grunts, but doesn't want to talk. I follow him down the stairs, waiting twice while he stops to catch his breath. He blows through his mouth, his lips pursed. "Just like Pop, only there's a sixty-year age gap," I think with some bitterness.

Lonnie sees him first. Matthew stands on the patio, surveying the three steps up to the back lawn. He attempts to climb the first one, but quickly finds that he's too weak, so retreats, presumably to think about the problem. None of the family move, or let on that they've seen him. They sit and chat, sipping wine and Harvey Wallbangers, waiting until he's ready. I could lift him up in a jiffy, but the message he's giving is clear. Ignoring everything but the task at hand, he lowers himself to his knees and, with great concentration, leaning heavily on his forearms, pulls first one leg and then the other laboriously up to the grass. Don, pretending to be happening by, helps him to his feet as casually as possible. A few more minutes elapse before his strength renews itself. He brushes the dirt from his pants. Now is the time for the entrance.

The family are careful not to overwhelm. They take in the changes privately — no one comments on his thinness or his colour, no one says how much older he seems. He's quiet and shy, and unusually polite. It is Mom who breaks the ice.

"Come here, you old turkey," she calls, holding out her arms. "Come and give Gramma a hug." Matthew throws his head back and laughs, relief written all over his face. Some things haven't changed, after all.

And so we settle into a routine of sorts, though nothing is like before. Matthew has little energy for any real activity, so books, puzzles and Transformers help to make up his day. He watches TV and videos by the hour, boundaries on such amusements having been greatly extended. His friends come to visit — Robert, Greg, Andrew, Nelson. Curious, quiet and shy at first, their self-consciousness soon disappears as they enter the world of He-Man together or share a colouring book.

Every day, three times a day, two white pills, enormous and bitter, are crushed between two teaspoons. This is tranexamic acid, a relatively new, relatively unknown drug that may help the blood in the abnormal vessels to clot. May. We try to mask the taste with milk, or sometimes apple juice, but the potion remains unpleasant, the texture gritty.

Matthew sits at the table, glass in hand, a dark scowl puckering his face.

"Come on, son," encourages Don. "Look, I'll take one of my pills first, then you swallow some of yours." He places a multivitamin on the back of his tongue and washes it down with some water.

"There. That was easy, wasn't it? Now it's your turn." Matt raises the glass to his lips. He holds his nose with the other hand, and takes the smallest of sips.

"Yuk," he says, screwing up his face and replacing the glass in disgust. And so the battle goes, on and on, three times a day, every day. . .

The prednisone is easier. The pills are smaller and more manageable. He quickly learns to wash them down with a large gulp of whatever he chooses. It becomes a ritual — this taking of the pills. And despite the hassle, it's important to us. It gives us some control. It's something we can "do." We know they're no more than chemical band-aids, but, strangely enough, with each little ceremony, our hope is renewed once more.

Each night we tuck him into bed, arranging him carefully against his pillows. His options have become more limited. He can no longer lie flat or on his left side. For some reason, which I don't fully understand, this makes him very breathless. The humidifier works constantly, moistening the air around him, helping to loosen the secretions in his lungs. I hear him in the bathroom in the small hours, coughing up phlegm and trying to clear his throat. The first few times, I tiptoe in to check. He is bent over the basin with the water running, and he makes it more than obvious that he'd rather be alone. This, I know, is his way of coping. I return to bed and weep. What else can one do?

Elizabeth is at school most days. I know who her teacher is, but that's as far as it goes. I drop her off for Brownies on Mondays, and for dancing on Wednesday afternoons. I no longer go into Marilyn's to watch her dance. It's suddenly irrelevant to know the fling, or to be able to assess her high-cuts. It is all so unimportant.

I sound like a parrot on the phone: "No, I'm sorry. I know you're short a Brownie leader, but. . ." "No, I'm sorry. I really can't help with the class outings at the moment. . ." "The Highland Dance Association? No, I'm sorry. My time is already spoken for. . ."

Our life revolves around Matthew, and Elizabeth, at seven, has to learn to "fit in" to suit our time and energy. There is no other way we can cope.

Our friends, however, provide the balance. Not just friends, either — acquaintances, too, offer to drive her to school, take her to the movies. There are unexpected party invitations, "new" invitations. There are letters through the mail-slot, only for her. "I'm knitting an outfit for your Cabbage Patch doll," writes one friend. "Please let me know which colours you like." There are cards decorated with dolls, kittens, puppies; there are strips of stickers: hearts, rainbows. They tell her that she's special, that she's loved.

Matthew and Elizabeth spend little time together, as both are busy in their separate worlds. They are quieter and gentler together — but the sibling bickering hasn't entirely disappeared.

"Elizabeth," I say, not infrequently, taking her aside. "You know that Matt is ill. You know he's been through a lot. Let's try to get on together, let's try and make each day count."

We take him to the hospital each week to be examined by Dr. Pritchard. She sometimes orders blood work, and sometimes X-rays. Occasionally a thoracentesis is needed to remove fluid from his chest. It never fails to amaze us that, after all he has been through, he loves to come back to the hospital. Don generally takes him in for these check-ups, and once the examination is over, they head down to I.C.U. to renew old friendships.

He's a very different child from the one we had known just months earlier. The sparkle has left his eyes; he is quiet and sedentary of necessity; and he has acquired wisdom and maturity far beyond his years.

Because he's too ill to go to school, we arrange for a tutor to come to the house several times a week. Mrs. Cowie's enthusiasm works wonders, and Matthew soon makes up for lost time. In mid-October, he appears to be stronger, and is adamant that he be treated normally. He joins his French-immersion grade one class, and we are delighted to find that he has a dedicated, sympathetic teacher. I tell Mme. Smith of his illness and the experiences of the past few months, and know immediately that all will be well at school.

Too soon, the mists of autumn rise from the bay and roll across the farmlands. Leaves in their thousands, orange and brown, fall to the lawns and driveways. The bright light of summer softens to gold, and the cold morning air hints of frosts to come. Pictures of cats, witches on broomsticks and ghosts adorn the fridge door. Halloween is here.

Six, it would seem, is the age for Dracula. "We've still got last year's mouse costume," I plead, but Matthew will not be deterred.

Our local department store has a large stock of Dracula kits. I rummage through them, hoping to find a kinder, more peaceful, less violent one than the ones I've seen. The search, of course, is in vain. Matthew will be a regular Dracula.

Come the big night, I help him with the transformation.

"You really don't need the white face-paint," I tell him, without belabouring the point. He draws black circles around his eyes, and blood — too lifelike — drips from his mouth. I help him fix the vampire teeth, implant a plastic mustache, and tie the black cloak at his throat.

"Wow, Matt!" I exclaim, laughing falsely. This is surely the thinnest, most ghoulish Dracula yet!

But Halloween doesn't last long. Within minutes, the vampire teeth are discarded, followed closely by the coarse plastic mustache. Matt leans forward, over the seat of his chair. His breathing is laboured, having been hampered by the accessories. He plucks reluctantly at the tie at his throat.

"Let's take it off for a minute, then," I say, and meet with no resistance.

The doorbell rings. It's Greg and his dad. Greg is a Dracula too, but all his trimmings are still intact. They head into the cold, wet night to join the throngs of trick-or-treaters. Matthew, Ken tells me later, makes it to the first three doors, then falls asleep, curled up on the back seat of the car.

I can hardly begin to explain the sadness of these days for me. It was Elisabeth Kübler-Ross who first talked about the "little deaths" that come with catastrophic illness. And every day we see them in our son. And every day, grief, which I'd always thought was a response to death, is present. We weep for what has been lost: the health of our child, and with it, an active, robust way of life. The mischievous gleam in his eye. His physical abilities, especially his love of bikes and ball games. His childhood innocence. Our dreams for the future.

And we weep in anticipation. Despite our never-ending hope, we cannot deny the serious faces and sombre words of the doctors. And yet, that's not entirely accurate. Denial is an important factor in the grief process, to be used as needed when reality is too painful to bear. We interpret the doctors' words to suit our ability to cope with them. We have to. We can't give up at this stage of the game.

In December, Matthew is re-admitted to Children's Hospital for a further thoracentesis, this time under general anaesthetic. His chest X-rays show that fluid is collecting again.

The results of the procedure are disappointing. The fluid has loculated and is impossible to extract. This has threatening implications: not only a further reduction in healthy lung tissue, but also an increased risk of infection. However, not all is gloom. Matthew is thrilled to be back in his "old" bed in I.C.U. The Child Life staff bring him games and activities. He loves the TV programs and videos, and especially the computer games. Miss B., one of the hospital teachers, brings school work to his bedside until he is able to attend the classroom.

He recognizes a number of the children in the non-acute area of I.C.U. from his previous admission, and renews his friendship with David, a delightful two-year-old dwarf who breathes by virtue of a tracheotomy. David's mom, Shirley, teaches us some sign language so that we can communicate with the child. "Say 'Happy Christmas' to Matthew, David," she encourages. The little guy is delighted to oblige. "No, no, David," his patient mom remonstrates. "That's 'Happy Elephant'! This is 'Happy Christmas.' Now try again."

No wonder Matt loves the hospital. This is a safe environment. Here, with help, he can meet any demands placed on him. He is cherished and pampered, and he loves his caregivers in return. He can forget his inability to run across the school field with his friends, or to play their games at recess. In the outside world, he is separated, different, handicapped. Here, he belongs. He has a visible network of support. Some of the younger children even rely on him for help and hugs. Here, he is King.

It's one day at a time at Children's, and during Christmas, each of those days is magical. Christmas trees and decorations adorn every corner and corridor. Busy volunteers sort and wrap the presents that flow in from beaming well-wishers. Mince tarts, Christmas cake and chocolates vie for space in the nursing stations. Good will abounds. At Christmas, a children's hospital acts as a magnet for anyone with charity to spare. Service clubs and sports teams masquerade as Santa's helpers. It's still a week before Christmas itself and Matt's loot is increasing daily. He's reluctant to come home. We can't, after all, compete with visits from the Vancouver Canucks hockey team and the B.C. Lions football team.

One evening Don and I reverse our usual routine. He is at the hospital. I am collapsed on the sofa, mindlessly watching the six o'clock news; Elizabeth is beside me, writing Christmas cards. The news is all predictable:

problems in the Middle East, political turmoil in Ottawa, appeals for food for the Vancouver Food Bank. There is nothing new. News anchor Bill Good Jr. is smiling broadly. "Santa was at B.C. Children's Hospital today," he says, "and our cameras went along." My eyes are riveted to the screen. I can hardly believe what I see. Santa is talking to Matthew. "And what would you like for Christmas, Matthew?" Matt is probably trying to think of something he has not already received. Believe me, it's a tough one! He finally settles on a Transformer, gives Santa a big hug, and the moment of stardom is over. Elizabeth and I beam at one another. There are perks, after all, in our unenviable situation, and this is definitely one.

The following day, Matthew comes home. There are only five more days until Christmas and we are determined to have a wonderful holiday. It's within our grasp if we just take one day at a time. Forget the future. Refuse to acknowledge that this may be his last Christmas. . .

His toys and puzzles cover the playroom floor. Elizabeth, too, is inundated with gifts from thoughtful friends. We are deeply grateful, not so much for the presents themselves as for the recognition of her feelings and needs.

Don and I could easily get away with being cheapskate Santas this year. A mandarin orange in the stocking toe, followed by a bag of marbles, batteries, candies, and other sundries. Easy! But we have needs, too. We continually guard against leaving room for regrets. Our need now is to give Matthew the best Christmas possible, a part of which is to choose the presents that he will most enjoy.

The first is a bike. It's yellow and black with the magic letters "BMX" inscribed on one of the bars. It matters not at all that it's from a garage sale and has clearly been revamped. Neither does it matter that, until now, he has been too weak for exercise. The bike represents a symbol of normalcy and our hopes for his future strength and happiness. The second gift is Optimus Prime — the ultimate Transformer. It's almost impossible to come by. Every young boy is convinced that he needs one. It graces the top of thousands of wish lists. With considerable difficulty, our friends, Ken and Sandy, track down what must surely be the last two in Vancouver. Matt's delight is our reward: our needs are met.

Christmas is spent largely with Don's family. A party atmosphere pervades all the activities. Matthew is with us — reason in itself for celebration. The richness of each moment is magnified, precious beyond words. A few days later we travel up to Kamloops to stay with our friends the Dregers. Cold, crisp, sunny days, sleigh rides across the fields, mulled wine and hot chocolate to warm body and soul. Log fires glowing from the hearth.

Children laughing together. Suppers to linger over. Wonderful friends willing to share our burdens.

Then back to the coast for New Year's Eve — bingo and videos with Don's family. Gramma helps Matthew with his bingo card. He wins a highly suspect number of games. We all have our needs.

Three minutes to midnight. On TV, the crowds roar from Times Square. Excited revellers wave and blow horns. The countdown begins.

I watch, mesmerized, gripped with fear. I don't want to move forward. The present is manageable and secure. The future holds shadows and uncertainty.

"Five. Four. Three. Two. One. It's 1986! Happy New Year, everybody."

The TV crowd goes wild, hugging and kissing. Arms crossed and holding hands, we join in "Auld Lang Syne" and hug each other in turn.

"Happy New Year, my Matthew," I whisper, planting a big kiss on his cheek. "Happy New Year."

Chapter Seven

Spring '86 is a time of great hope.

For whatever reason, Matthew seems better. The sparkle has returned to his eyes, he is coughing less, he is riding his new bike. He is back at school — not merely one day here, one day there, but every day, just like normal kids. He has joined Beavers again. Each Monday, he dons the brown uniform jacket and blue cotton hat before picking at his supper.

"Sharing! Sharing! Sharing!" we joke, hands held up to imitate paws. And he laughs and laughs. He's eating more, too — not much more, but it's definitely an improvement — and surely that's a sign that we're winning.

"I don't need to see him every week now," Sheila tells us halfway through January. "Once every two weeks, so long as he's well, will be just fine."

Our prayers must be being answered. God knows, there are enough people down on their knees on Matthew's behalf. He seems to be on everybody's prayer list, not only here, but in England as well. "Our minister prayed for Matthew again on Sunday," Mum tells me during one of our frequent transatlantic calls, "and I know he's often remembered at both John's and Helen's churches." Don's mom also has a hotline to the sky, and her contact with a spiritual group down in the States has ensured supplication from that country, too. It's obvious that God is being bombarded.

"Maybe he'll make Matthew well just to get us off his back," Don jokes, trusting that whoever is up there has at least a small sense of humour.

We ease ourselves gradually into normal-life activities. Don starts work on his nets and resumes his pursuits in the politics of fishing. I, at last, find some much-needed energy, and for the first time in months, apply it to the neglected house and garden. I take up aerobics in a modest way, and, session by session, am able to feel the difference. Weary muscles slowly respond, and my lethargy, so draining, begins to dissolve.

And Elizabeth — suddenly I notice her more. We have time to talk, to laugh, to share. "How's school going?" "Do you like your teacher?" "Who are your best friends?" Questions so basic, but missing for such a long while. Yes, suddenly there's room, and she has edged into focus once more.

As winter softens into spring, we dare to hope that Matthew will indeed get well. God, we reason, is intervening. Maybe the bitter white pills are working, after all. Perhaps, just maybe . . . This is indeed a time of great hope.

I read voraciously — "searching," I believe it's called. It has become a necessity, as vital to me as eating or sleeping. I browse for hours in bookstores, hunting for anything that will help us cope, that will shed a little light on our experiences. My hunger for understanding is insatiable; books lie in piles by my bed. There never seems to be enough time to devour their wisdom. Two books in particular, *Teach Only Love* and *Creative Visualization*, are always close at hand. They help me escape from the terror of reality, and teach me that while I cannot change my circumstances, I can change my responses and attitudes to them. This knowledge is invaluable.

Spring break is upon us. Not wanting to venture too far from the hospital, we book a few days at Port Ludlow, a quiet resort in northern Washington.

"You'll love it," Geraldine tells us. "It's not too far, and it's well set up for families."

The morning is clear and sunny. Cases, bags and an assortment of favourite toys are stacked and waiting in the downstairs hall. Matthew is in the bathroom, coughing over the basin as he always does first thing.

"Dad!" he suddenly yells, as loudly as his disease will permit. The urgency in his voice brings Don and me to the bathroom door in seconds. We stare in horror at the basin.

"It's just a little blood," Don tells him calmly, rinsing the damning evidence away. "It's nothing to worry about, son. The doctors said this might happen."

"How will we know if the disease is progressing?" we had asked Sheila some months earlier.

"We don't know for sure," she had told us, "but we think there'll be bleeding into his lungs. It'll probably show up as blood in his sputum."

Don's eyes meet mine above our small son's head, mirroring the unspoken anguish my face must surely reveal.

"Just keep a good eye on him," Sheila advises, returning our phone call promptly. "There's really nothing we can do, but do bring him in if you're worried."

We react by rebelling, refusing to accept that the "good time" is over — that Matthew is out of remission. We pack the van and flee, keeping to plans already made, as if somehow, by acting normally, we can make it all right again.

We should've realized that we couldn't escape. Our sadness and torment travel with us, colouring each scene. Memories of our holiday: Matt, unable to walk up a slope . . . Matt, exhausted after hitting one tennis ball . . . Matt, watching us swim from the side of the pool . . . Matt, ashen-faced, fishing from the pier . . .

Shortly after we return from our nightmare, a friend suggests the Mayo Clinic. "Leave no stone unturned," she says, "leave no room for regrets." We leap at the suggestion, desperate for anything that might help us, frantic for something to hold onto. Hope has come in many guises. The Mayo Clinic is about to join the list.

The morning of Saturday, April 26 is bright and sunny and full of the aromas and sounds of spring. It's my birthday. I'm forty today. Forty! Is that all?

It promises to be memorable. Not exactly what I would have chosen for my "big four-oh," mind you, but memorable nonetheless. Today we fly down to the Mayo Clinic. An appointment has been made, airline tickets bought, and our bags packed. Mike and Diane, Don's nephew and his wife, are here to look after Elizabeth while we are away.

Medical reports, X-rays, a biopsy slide, medications. We check and recheck that we have everything. Our plan is to drive the 180 kilometres to Seattle and fly from there, first to Minneapolis and finally to Rochester.

I don't see it at first. I'm so busy waving goodbye and making sure that Matthew is all right in the back seat, that it quite passes me by. But all of a sudden, my gaze is drawn up to the visor, and there it is: the most beautiful long-stemmed red rose you could ever imagine.

"Oh, hon, is this for me?" Don is wearing his sheepish look, which defies all description. He extracts a tape from his pocket and slips it into the tape-deck.

"Happy birthday, hon. It's made up of some of our favourite songs," he explains, looking more sheepish than ever. They are, without exception, love songs, beautiful and poignant.

"Thanks, hon. You couldn't have given me anything that would be more special."

"Mom."

"Yes, Matthew?"

"Tell me again why we're goin' on this trip?"

"Well, the Mayo Clinic is supposed to be the best in the world, son. The best doctors, the best equipment, the best everything. We're hoping that they may have seen your illness before, and be able to offer some other treatments."

The explanation suffices and he returns to his world of Transformers and books.

We stop for brunch halfway to Seattle. The restaurant is crowded and the service unhurried. We are left with barely enough time to get to Sea-Tac Airport, and curse ourselves for adding to our problems.

"Rochester, New York or Rochester, Minnesota?" the ticket agent asks. "You'd be surprised how many people make mistakes on that one!"

The flight to Minneapolis appears to be unremarkable. Matt sleeps for almost the entire journey. His pallor disturbs me, but it has done so often before. I am just thankful that he is resting. On the second leg of the trip, from Minneapolis to Rochester, the plane bumps and tosses constantly. Someone behind us jokes about tornadoes in this area. We don't appreciate their sense of humour! We fly at low altitude for the thirty-minute journey, which gives us panoramic views of the lovely Minnesota countryside below. Matt, awake and alert, enjoys it too. His eyes are no longer glassy and his skin looks less like putty.

The air is hot and sultry and, in the distance, the sky rumbles angrily. "We've had a lot of tornado warnings lately," our cab driver mentions nonchalantly. Don and I exchange glances — just what we needed to hear!

Rochester, home of the Mayo Foundation, is an extremely pleasant surprise. We had, for some reason, expected a large and dirty city enveloping the clinics and labs, renowned the world over. But not at all. The town is relatively small, having, our cabbie tells us, a population of 60,000 permanent residents. The streets are wide and spacious and the buildings are clean. The taxi deposits us and our baggage at the entrance to the Kahler Hotel, an elegant establishment in the centre of town that was recommended to us by a friend. We've already made reservations. Matt sinks into a plush armchair while we wait.

"Your room is ready for you, sir. We'll bring an extra bed in for your son. Just one night? Very good, sir."

The room is not particularly large, but it's comfortable, and decorated with quiet good taste. A colourful bouquet of flowers stands on the table, blending perfectly with its surroundings. It is several minutes before we realize that they do not come with the price of the room. A small card hides amongst the foliage. It wishes me "Happy Birthday" and sends love and best wishes from good friends in Tsawwassen. Suddenly, home seems closer, the week ahead less threatening.

As soon as we are refreshed and fed, we set out to explore something of our surroundings. Across the road from the Kahler, and dominating the area, is a beautiful white multi-storied building which we quickly learn is Mayo Clinic itself. We also discover that in the immediate centre of Rochester there are eleven other buildings that are part of the clinic or affiliated with it in some way. Most of these are linked by large lighted pedestrian underpasses, allowing easy passage from one to the other. The Kahler Hotel, along with some of the city's other major establishments, is also connected to the clinic by this means.

It's obvious that Rochester's facilities are geared, almost totally, toward the needs of people who, like ourselves, require its medical services. There are numerous hotels and motels clustered within easy reach of the centre. Wheelchairs can be borrowed or rented without difficulty, and the sidewalks were designed with their presence in mind. Drug stores and medical supplies abound. Church groups reach out to those in need of support and encouragement. It seems that everything is orchestrated to make life as simple as possible for the clinic's patients and their families.

The Kahler is a treat, but a little too fancy for our needs and our bank account. Also, we require a kitchenette and a separate bedroom for Matthew. He is restless at night, occasionally sitting bolt upright in his sleep in order to breathe more easily. Periodically, he attempts to clear his throat of stagnant phlegm or unclog his bronchial tubes of stifling secretions. I am often awakened by the ominous sounds of his coughing, and am familiar with my own reactions — fear and anger, and sadness of an indescribable intensity. So a separate bedroom is essential, not so much to protect Matthew from our sounds as to, in some measure, protect us from his. Survival is the name of the game.

The next day Don scouts the area and finds a motel tailor-made to our requirements. Soldiers Field 4th Street Motel, an older two-storey building, is a short walk from the clinic and the centre of town. Our unit has both a kitchenette and a separate bedroom. We settle in and prepare for whatever the week will bring.

It's amazing to us that the Mayo Clinic is situated in a farming area in Minnesota, for there could hardly be a more unlikely setting. Why, we wonder, is it not in New York, Chicago or Los Angeles? We don't have to look far to find the answers. The motel lobby holds a wealth of information for tourists; among the many brochures are several that tell the history of the celebrated medical facilities. We learn that the Mayo Clinic grew from the medical practice of a country doctor, William Worrall Mayo, who moved to Rochester in 1863. His sons, William and Charles, assisted him during their boyhood, and later, as doctors themselves, joined him in the family practice. They were not only skilled and enthusiastic but also tireless in their pursuit of knowledge and innovative ideas. They eventually attracted international attention, and doctors and scientists from around the world travelled great distances for the privilege of watching their surgical techniques and learning from them. They soon outgrew their practice and, of necessity, invited other doctors to join them in what was to become the world's first private group medical practice. Specialists in many fields complemented their medical skills, and they formed teams of experts, which then required further organization. The system developed to coordinate the activities of physicians and patients, the training of medical specialists, and the growth of medical research is what we know as the Mayo Clinic today.

By Monday morning the heat and threatening winds have subsided and, thank God, the tornado warning is over for the present. We don't want to be wimps, but we're not accustomed to tornadoes and certainly need no more problems at the moment! The change in weather is dramatic. Cold air has moved in to replace yesterday's sauna, and grey clouds hang low. We are up early, anxious to be punctual and well presented on our first day. Matthew can't walk all of the three blocks to the clinic, so Don and I take turns carrying him. The sidewalks are filled with hundreds of clinic employees hurrying to their work. The general impression is one of women in their twenties and thirties, most dressed in white or pastel uniforms. These, we guess, are the nurses, receptionists, lab and X-ray technicians. The well-dressed men sporting briefcases we take to be doctors, and the smartly dressed women with similar hand baggage must be doctors too, or possibly secretaries. It's much easier to pick out the patients. Some ride in wheelchairs or lean on canes or crutches. Some are supported by family or friends. There is often at least one clue to connect them to a file in the Registration Office: poor colour, laboured breathing, Down's syndrome, irregular gait, rasping cough, physical abnormalities of every kind. No, there are no prizes for picking out the patients.

The clinic reception area is expansive, clean and surprisingly peaceful despite the hundreds of people gathered here. We report to the registration desk, where a file is opened for Matthew.

"Paediatrics is on E9," we are told. "Do borrow a wheelchair if you'd like to. They're by the main doors. The elevators are to your left."

Matthew clambers into the wheelchair and we join the crowd of people waiting for the elevators. The Paediatrics waiting area is empty, but three nurses are busy at the front desk. We introduce ourselves and fill out the necessary forms. Matthew shows a Transformer to one of the nurses and tries to start a conversation. The nurse, however, has little time to socialize.

"Take a seat in the waiting room, please. Dr. O'Connell will see you shortly."

The wait seems interminable, but is merely good practice for the week ahead!

At long last it is our turn. Dr. O'Connell greets us at the nurses' station. Our welcome could not be warmer: he is the gracious host and we are the guests. He leads us down a long hallway and into a brightly lit examining room where we settle ourselves into a comfortable sofa. Matthew spies some toys of interest and kneels to inspect them more closely. Dr. O'Connell sits down at his desk and thumbs through our file. Sheila Pritchard has produced a painstaking medical report on Matthew, and it is this which commands all of his attention.

We know little of this man who we hope can provide some solutions to our problems. He is somewhere in his mid-fifties and strikes us as immensely likable. As are all the physicians practising at the Mayo, he is here by invitation — and in order to be invited, he must have had an excellent reputation. He peers intently through half-moon glasses resting on the tip of his nose. We watch for clues as he reads the details of our son's illness, hanging on every raised eyebrow, each almost imperceptible shake of the head. Sheila's detailed medical report is a luxury and Dr. O'Connell comments on its thoroughness.

"It's most helpful to have a report like this," he tells us. "Many patients arrive at the clinic without their G.P.'s knowledge or blessing. As a consequence, we have nothing more to go on than the patient's own interpretation of his or her medical history."

Dr. O'Connell, like all the Mayo doctors, is on salary and free from the pressures of having to hurry through a long patient list. As a result, there is no rush, no sense of urgency, no sounds of the next patient being shown into an adjoining examining room. We soon learn that thoroughness and meticulous attention to detail are never sacrificed for speed. After what seems like an eternity, Dr. O'Connell slowly puts down the report.

"Climb up on here, Matthew. Let's have a look at you." We have sat through numerous physicals in the past eight months. All have been thorough, but none more so than this one. Finally released, Matthew slides down from the table and heads for the nurses' station.

Dr. O'Connell writes for several minutes. Eventually, he puts down his pen, but still says nothing. He removes his glasses with one hand and with the other slowly rubs his eyes in a way that suggests it has already been a long, hard day. At last, he speaks.

"Matthew's case certainly appears to be both complex and serious, but we'll try not to make any judgement calls at this stage. What I plan to do is to talk to my colleagues. I will be consulting with a number of other doctors, each one a specialist in his own field. They will see Matthew and yourselves, and between us we will order all necessary tests and X-rays. The nurses will arrange the appointments for you and I will see you periodically and will endeavour to keep you up to date."

There are no false hopes, no magic words.

For the next five days our world is a succession of consultants, waiting rooms, X-rays, scans and blood tests. By Friday we are navigating the underground passageways like veterans. We could pass as novice tour guides for the labs and diagnostic buildings. Complex medical terminology rolls off our tongues with ease, and Matthew is by now, of course, right at home in the nurses' station!

It is late on Friday afternoon when we finally meet again with Dr. O'Connell. He tells us that there are still more tests needed in order to complete the medical picture. In a now familiar gesture, he removes his glasses and rubs his eyes. He appears to be very weary. He reaches in vain for the right words; but there are none. The raw truth will have to suffice.

"The original diagnosis appears to be accurate, though there may be considerable involvement of the lymph system too. A lymph angiogram has been scheduled for Monday morning in order to determine the degree of complicity." He pauses again, as though to choose his words with care.

"Your son's illness is extremely rare," he starts. "Our consultants have seen very few cases of this disease, and certainly none as diffuse as Matthew's. Most of the patients were children, and all have died. The options for treatment are extremely limited. The only suggestion which would be anything less than a band-aid is a heart/lung transplant, which is, of course, precariously aggressive."

"How did it start, Dr. O'Connell?" Don asks the question that has plagued us both for months. "Is it hereditary? Is it something we did?" The doctor shakes his head.

"As far as we know, there is no genetic factor involved. And," he stresses, "it is nothing that you did. There are no answers as to why the disease should have started in Matthew, though the X-ray on Monday may throw more light on the question. It is a fluke. A chance in millions. It just happened."

There is little more to add for the moment.

"Thank you, Dr. O'Connell, and have a good weekend yourself."

Matt hugs the nurses goodbye. He has "helped" them for the past three days and is duly rewarded with "Get-Along Gang" stickers and magnets.

That night we wait until Matthew settles to sleep, then silently weep together. Mayo Clinic was a hope — a small one, admittedly, but a hope nonetheless. What will we hold onto now?

On Saturday we sleep in late and then saunter around the shops. We find the library and spend a short time browsing through books and magazines. In a gloomy upstairs room a handful of children and parents are waiting for the start of a film. We join their numbers, but an old, faulty version of *Johnny Appleseed* has no hope of competing with modern cartoons, and

Matt's attention wanders after the first few minutes.

The weekend is warm and sunny, so the next day we decide to explore more of Rochester. We push Matthew in a rented wheelchair and head away from the centre of town. After about a mile, we reach the enormous complex comprising St. Mary's Hospital, one of two hospitals affiliated with the clinic. Both Rochester Methodist and St. Mary's are private hospitals with medical staffs composed entirely of Mayo Clinic physicians. On the way home we pass a park in which several children of about Matt's age are laughing and playing on the swings. They pause in their games and stare at the boy in the wheelchair. He watches them in silence but carefully avoids their eyes. By the time we return to the motel, he's decidedly cranky. I can't say I blame him.

On Monday morning Don takes Matthew for the lymph angiogram. It's basically an X-ray, but the preparation is unpleasant and painful. Radioactive dye is injected into lymphatic vessels between the toes, and in turn shows up in the lymphatic system. Matthew is miserable. He has had enough. He wants to go home. No more needles, no more tests, no more waiting. It's at this point that we learn he must have a thoracentesis this afternoon. It's the last test, and an important one. Matt, of course, has had them before and knows they are no fun. Don takes him aside and tells him the bad news as positively as he is able.

Matt listens in silence. His large eyes flash angrily and brim with tears. He gets up and, back erect, walks briskly to the washroom. Don is at the end of his tether. He follows his son into the washroom area and waits by the basin. He waits and waits. He can see the small black shoes and grey socks under the door. Matthew is simply standing there trying to deal with his misery alone. Fortunately, one can look at washroom walls only so long, and he finally emerges. He is obviously shaken by what he sees: Don is crying. His tall, strong, loving Dad is actually crying.

"It's all right, Dad. I'll have the tap. It's no problem. Don't cry, Dad." He takes Don's hand and hugs him comfortingly. He assumes the role of caregiver. He is six years old, after all, and his courage and strength are needed. "All right now, Dad? Please don't cry."Tuesday, May 6.

The tests and X-rays are all completed. The evidence is in. All that remains is for the verdict to be delivered. We're not expecting good news. The day promises to be full of pain. Don and I remind each other that this will certainly be the case and we prepare psychologically, as best we can, for what we must hear. Matthew is pleased for another opportunity to be with his friends the nurses. He slides onto the stool next to Terri, his favourite, determined to make the best of their last day together.

Dr. Telander, the paediatric surgeon, sees us first, and explains the findings of the lymph angiogram. There is definitely an acquired blockage of the thoracic duct. Without drainage to the liver, the lymph has sought other routes and the disease process has been launched. Corrective surgery is not feasible; the only option that might be explored is a heart/lung transplant. This is a new and uncharted form of treatment, but it's a possibility. Dr. Telander tells us that he has already discussed Matthew's case with a Dr. Jamieson of the University of Minnesota. If we wish, an appointment can be arranged to see him before we leave for Canada. We do wish! It's a lifeline. Another source of hope.

"Thank you, Dr. Telander," we say.

Dr. O'Connell greets us like old friends and motions to the familiar sofa. He chooses his words with great care, but there is no easy way to tell us the conclusion of their findings. The diagnosis is, without doubt, diffuse pulmonary haemangioma and lymphangioma. He tells us that both of the lungs and surrounding structures are involved. Corrective surgery is not feasible, as we already know. The disease is slowly progressing and will gradually use up all vital lung tissue. Matthew's prognosis is very poor.

"How long do you think he has, Dr. O'Connell?" Don's voice sounds strange and distant. The doctor removes his glasses and rubs his eyes, as we knew he would. There is a long silence. My initial dread has given way to a numbness which I know and welcome.

"It's difficult to know for certain," he answers finally. "The disease is so rare that we have little to go on." He pauses again.

"We could guess at probably anything from a few months to a few years. Looking at his present state of health, possibly two years."

There is another silence. Two years? Maybe less? All feeling has gone, thank God.

"And how is he likely to die, Dr. O'Connell?" I hear a voice much like my own ask the unthinkable.

The doctor ponders the possibilities for what seems like a lifetime. And then, "Again, one cannot know for certain. But it is my opinion that he will, after some respiratory distress, have a peaceful death. It is likely that he will become hypoxic — short of oxygen — go into a coma and die in his sleep."

We rise to leave. We have our facts straight and the certain knowledge that no stone has been left unturned. Now, if only the numbness will last we can exit with some semblance of dignity.

Dr. O'Connell clasps our hands warmly.

"I'll pray for Matthew and for your family," he tells us. "We'll keep in touch. I'll be very interested to hear what Dr. Jamieson can offer."

Matthew hugs and kisses first his nurses and then his doctor.

"Thank you," we say. "Thank you for everything."

Our favourite restaurant is a couple of blocks away. Matthew can just manage it on foot as long as we walk slowly and stop several times to rest. We are in no hurry anyway. The restaurant is housed in a wooden, high-ceilinged structure and the scent of natural wood is a first impression — even more dominant than the wonderful aromas wafting from the kitchen. The waiter is beginning to know us.

"A carafe of the house white?" he asks, and returns with it promptly. The wine is cold and soothing. We both gulp down our first glass, anticipating the temporary relief it will bring. Matthew studiously examines the red and white checkered tablecloth, and fiddles with the children's menu. We are totally unprepared for his question.

"Can the doctors do anything for me?" he asks, still looking down and carefully avoiding our eyes. We're taken off-guard. There's been no preparation, no rehearsal.

"No, son," Don tells him. "They were able to give us a lot of information about your illness, but they don't have a cure. However, we're going to see another doctor on Thursday and he may well be able to help."

The bowed head is immobile. Tears would be appropriate, or even a tantrum. He has every right to be both angry and afraid. But Matthew does nothing — just sits and stares blankly at the pattern of the tablecloth.

"Are you disappointed, fella?" I finally ask.

"Yes," he nods and immediately falls asleep, his head cradled in his arms, resting on the table.

Minneapolis is a ninety-mile drive from Rochester, and the following day we rent a car and start out on our journey. The sky is a brilliant blue and the air feels warm and balmy. We cruise through mile after mile of open, rolling, green countryside — it could be a delightful trip under different circumstances.

Minneapolis, our destination, is the largest city in Minnesota. It's separated from St. Paul only by the Mississippi River, and together they are known as the Twin Cities.

The city itself is extremely large and sprawling. We soon realize that we are hopelessly lost, and wind up as reluctant participants in their rush hour! It is with considerable trouble that we locate a suitable motel, and settle in for the night.

The University of Minnesota Hospital is situated along East River Road at Harvard Street. We know little about this institution, but several factors give us confidence. A referral from the Mayo speaks highly of the hospital's reputation, and the very existence of a major transplant unit indicates expertise and equipment of the highest calibre. The hospital can also boast, among its past and present staff, surgeons whose names have gone down in history for their contributions to medical science. Of them all, Christian Barnard is perhaps the most famous.

Shortly after 1:30 p.m. we park the car and follow the signs for "cardiothoracic surgery." The buildings are austere — definitely not designed with beauty in mind! One has a feeling of being immersed in cold, grey concrete. It is stark and unfriendly. Foreboding.

"Well, the good news is that it isn't a fire hazard," Don jokes. No one laughs. We're nervous and in need of comfort. There are no silly giraffes painted on the walls here, no cows eating daisies, no piped music. I am suddenly sick with fear. What if there is no hope? What if they turn us down?

The receptionist is everything that our surroundings lack. Friendly and warm, she puts us both at ease and she and Matt are soon deep in conversation.

"Well, I've heard of a girl in every port, but this is a case of a nurse in every office." Don grins. The receptionist plays along, and Matthew, certain of another conquest, beams.

Dr. Stuart Jamieson appears at the door. I had expected an older man — someone intense, anxious, rushing around in doctor's greens from one operating room to another. This man looks to be about our age (what have we been doing with life while he's been learning to transplant hearts?). He is tall and handsome, with a relaxed, affable manner that lends itself to casual conversation. Born in Africa, trained in London, England, he has recently come from Stanford University in California to head the cardiac transplant team here.

"How many heart/lung transplants have actually been performed?" Don asks, finally getting down to specifics.

"About a hundred and fifty, to date," he tells us. "They've mainly been in the States and England, and the success rate has been very encouraging. Over 70 percent have survived and are doing relatively well. I understand you have some X-rays for me to look at?" Don produces the large brown envelope and Dr. Jamieson turns and studies the ominous pictures for several minutes.

Don and I make a pretence of relaxing in our seats, but pretence is all it is. Don's knuckles are white as he grips the arm of his chair. He gnaws at the skin around his nails on the other hand, as though he has not seen food for a week. As for me, I have developed a nervous twitch in my leg and cannot keep it still. It might be funny at any other time, but right now, too much hangs in the balance. What if a transplant isn't possible? What if the answer is no? What if this tall, attractive man has to turn around and tell us: "Sorry, it can't be done"? What then? How could we possibly cope with getting home? What would we tell Matthew? That he's dying? That we'll make the best of the time we have left? We desperately need some hope. Please say yes, Dr. Jamieson.

"I'd like a colleague to see these." Stuart Jamieson is already dialling a number. "Would you excuse me one moment?" He talks briefly into the phone, and within a matter of minutes, the door opens and a fresh-faced, bespectacled man enters. Introductions are made but I'm too busy trying to control my wayward twitch to catch his name. Don and I resume our seats while the two specialists examine the X-rays. I can't understand their analysis, but it takes them only a short time to reach a consensus.

"Sorry, I must dash, Stuart; I've got a two-thirty appointment to keep." He turns to Don and me. "It was very nice meeting you," he says, as Don and I search his face, in vain, for clues. "Have a good journey home." The door closes behind him.

Stuart Jamieson sits and faces us.

"Well, this is certainly an unusual case," he starts. "Matthew's operation would be rather more complicated than average, not only because of the disease, but because he has scarring from previous surgery." He pauses, scrutinizing the X-rays once more. "Anyway, there is no big rush to perform such a risky procedure on him at this stage; ideally we like no more than a six-month prognosis." He smiles — a big, relaxed, handsome smile. "Let's keep in touch and see how he does."

We are totally unprepared for the events of our trip home. We fly back by a different route — from Minneapolis to Denver and then from Denver to Seattle. About halfway through the first leg of the flight, Matt complains of nausea and stomach pains. He has reverted to the colour of putty once more. His breathing is shallow, his nails are blue, and his eyes have a distant, glazed expression. Suddenly he vomits. Mucous and sputum project from his nose and mouth. He doesn't seem to care — he is obviously too ill. Were he in hospital, the respiratory team would be on their way. But he's not in hospital, he's 30,000 feet in the air. Momentarily dizzy from terror, I imagine his sluggish breathing becoming slower and slower . . .

"Ladies and gentlemen," the Captain drawls, "we're nearing our destination of Denver, but the tower has just informed us that there's a forty-five- minute delay. We apologize for this but we'll be in a holding pattern until we receive permission to land. We hope you've had a pleasant flight and will fly with us again. Thank you."

I flag down a passing flight attendant. "Excuse me, our son is very ill. Could we have some oxygen?"

We have to try something. Oxygen will either help considerably or, because of the nature of his illness, make matters worse. If this doesn't work, I'm thinking, we'll have to request a priority landing.

Glancing at Matthew, the attendant quickly realizes the gravity of the situation.

"Cindy," she calls to another woman, "I need some help."

A cylinder of oxygen appears as if by magic. Within seconds, the two attendants have connected Matthew to it, a white mask covering his nose and mouth.

"Tell the captain, Cindy," the older woman commands, and Cindy hurries towards the cockpit. It occurs to me that a touch of drama is possibly a welcome change from serving meals and discharging pillows.

Suddenly we've become centre-stage.

"Oxygen . . . little boy . . . ill . . ." I hear whispers all around us and see the curious faces peering from every direction. An offensively cheerful lady sitting immediately in front of us peers over the seat. Quite clearly, she has no measure of the true situation.

"Bless him!" she purrs, "Got a little airsick, has he? Isn't he sweet!" She means well, but it is all I can do not to scream at her, filling her in on every detail, every thoracentesis, every blood test, every radical change in his brief life. I could finally vent my anger and fear by a brief summary of his pathetic prognosis. Airsick, my eye!

Matthew is very still. We watch him intently, monitoring every breath. Don's face is as pale as his son's and I suspect that I don't look much better!

We're lucky this time. Within minutes Matthew improves dramatically. His skin returns to its customary pallor and the vacant look recedes from his eyes. He even manages a weak smile.

"That was pretty rough on you, fella," I tell him.

"What was?"

"Well, you know, when you were so sick."

"Sick. When was I sick?"

"Nothing, guy. Glad you're better now." He truly doesn't remember. There probably wasn't enough oxygen to his brain. I shake my head in wonderment, thankful for small mercies.

Denver Airport is chaos. Dozens of planes are stacked up, circling over the city. Each incoming flight is late. Consequently, hundreds of people have missed connections and need to have their flights rebooked. We aren't exempt. We're frightened at the thought of taking Matthew on another plane and consider driving home instead; but a long car journey is also a poor prospect. I decide that on the trip to Seattle, our flight attendant will be forewarned. We can't afford any mistakes. Don has grave doubts about this strategy, but I insist.

The 747 is full and ready for take-off.

"Excuse me," I start, "we may need oxygen on the journey. Our little boy has a chest illness and was rather sick on the last flight." Obviously alarmed, the young flight attendant calls to a colleague in the next section. Flustered and carrying an armload of pillows, the older attendant listens while I repeat the story.

"We just wanted to make certain that there was oxygen available. Our son needed it on the last flight," Don explains. "It probably won't happen again, but we thought we should check."

She asks a few more questions, glances at Matthew, and hurries away. The heavy front door slams shut. The whine of the engines tell us that departure is imminent.

"This is the child," the second flight attendant nods towards Matthew. Her companion, a red-faced man somewhere in his mid-forties, is clearly agitated. He checks his watch and signals to another crew member who holds a telephone to her ear.

"Do you have a doctor's note?" the purser asks crisply.

"We didn't realize it was necessary." There is more than a hint of impatience in Don's voice. "The last flight was the first time this happened."

"I can't let you travel with an ill child," he apologizes. "I can't take that responsibility. If we have to make an emergency landing, it would cost the airline thousands of dollars and cause many of the passengers to miss their connecting flights." Don casts a withering glance in my direction and shakes his head in frustration.

"But how will we get home?" I ask, tears stinging my eyes. Matthew looks up from his Transformer. It's impossible to know what he thinks of this latest drama. It's all too much for the purser.

"Wait," he says, "we'll call the doctor. What's the boy's condition called?"

There are whispers around us again. Curious faces glance discreetly in our direction, not without sympathy. For others, it is yet another hold-up, another hassle. The wait seems interminable. Finally, the bulky entrance door reopens and, escorted by the purser, the doctor arrives, flushed and panting, at our seats.

"Pulmonary what?" he asks, after listening to a brief description of Matthew's problems.

"Haemangiomatosis, pul-mo-na-ry hae-man-gi-o-ma-to-sis." Don is beside himself. I can recognize the signs. He has had enough of this circus. Please don't say anything, Don, I'm thinking. We just want to get home.

The phone rings and is quickly answered by the purser. He talks fast, glaring steadily in our direction. The flustered doctor has had enough, too!

"You can fly this time," he concedes, "but next time, you must have a medical certificate." He sprints down the aisle, nods at the purser, and disappears through the doorway.

Don's eyes bore into mine above the head of our son. No words are spoken. None are needed.

Matthew is quiet on the flight, but fortunately suffers no further trauma. What relief we feel on reaching Seattle! Solid ground never felt so good!

"Never again, Don. Never again."

Don merely nods. He looks older than I had realized.

We retrieve the van from Sea-Tac parking lot and head north on Interstate 5. Matthew, propped up on the back seat, is asleep in minutes. My birthday rose is still in the visor. Its crimson petals, once fresh and full of life, are dry and fragile and tinged with brown. Don slips my tape into the deck and poignant melodies break through the silence of our misery.

"And who, who could have seen this coming, and dream it would happen to us?" Juice Newton croons. We weep together, sharing a box of tissues. I can't describe the depth of our pain.

It's early evening when we pass the Peace Arch and cross the border into Canada. The sky is clear and the majestic North Shore mountains rise above Vancouver in the distance. An orange sun flirts with the waters of Boundary Bay.

"What now, Mom?" Matthew has awakened and, like us, is thinking ahead.

"Oh, back to school, fella, so long as you're feeling OK. We'll go and see Dr. Pritchard next week. She'll want to know what the Mayo doctors have said."

What now? he's asking! What now, indeed.

Chapter Eight

Sheila Pritchard looks tired. She is eight months pregnant, and is also carrying a full workload in the Department of Oncology and Haematology. She listens attentively to our report from the Mayo Clinic. Dr. O'Connell has promised to send a written report to her within a few days, but for the moment, our interpretation must suffice. Matthew has left her office and is playing with the games in the day-treatment room. He always leaves when he's going to be the topic of conversation.

"So a transplant is the only possibility." Sheila is thinking aloud. This is no surprise to her, merely confirmation.

"In that case we need to get him into the best physical condition possible." She reaches for his chart and studies it for several minutes.

"Hmm, his weight is still twenty kilos. He hasn't put on any weight since the surgery last fall."

"We can't get him to eat," Don interjects. "He has no appetite. We seem to have tried everything."

"How would you feel about bringing him into hospital and building him up by nasogastric feeding? We'd insert a plastic tube into his nose and down into his stomach, and then feed him with special high-calorie formulas."

"Wonderful," Don and I respond together. The very thought of his thin body growing bigger and stronger brings joy.

"I'll try and get a bed for him right away." Sheila adds, "Plan for tomorrow, all being well."

We are delighted to be doing something positive in what appears to be an almost hopeless situation. Matt, too, is pleased with the news. Being in hospital means being special and fitting in at the same time.

The next day, May 14, Matthew is admitted to a four-bed room on 3B, and the nasogastric feedings are started the following evening. The plan is for Matt to eat regular meals during the day and to be fed the special formula at night. We can hardly wait to see more flesh on his spindly arms and bony bottom.

A few days later, there is a new patient in Matt's room. He lies on his bed, a tall, good-looking boy with dark brown eyes and hair. A pleasant lady with an English accent hovers around him, wearing the standard glazed expression of the newly-initiated 3B parent.

"We've just found out that Tony has leukaemia," she tells us, before any introductions have been made. "It's come as an awful shock, even though I'm a nurse, and it had vaguely crossed my mind — what with the pain in his hip, and he was so tired. But you don't think this kind of thing will ever happen to you or your family, do you? I'm Katie by the way. Katie Di Iuorio. This is Tony, of course, and Marcus here has already made friends with Matthew." Marcus is sitting on the edge of Matt's bed. He is a younger version of his teenage brother: the same dark eyes and hair, the same fine features.

"I'm a Katie, too. And English. And a nurse." We laugh in astonishment, managing to avoid acknowledging our ultimate bond.

Tony is calm but incredulous. He appears to be dazed, ill at ease with his newfound knowledge. Like his mother, he has a great need to talk.

"The doctor told us all about it," he starts. "If you're going to get leukaemia, then this is the best one to have. The survival rate is pretty high, though the treatment doesn't sound too good." Tony continues his monologue, regurgitating every medical detail that comes to mind.

In the days ahead, Tony and Matthew, in spite of their nine-year age difference, become soulmates. They seem to share a special understanding of their vulnerable situation, and they quickly form a deep friendship. They spend hours playing cards together or playing with Tony's computer and computer games. When Tony starts his chemotherapy treatments and begins to feel desperately ill, Matt is attentive to his every need.

"Is he going to die?" he asks a nurse on one of Tony's especially grim days. Reassured, he returns to his bed and keeps a watchful eye on his pal. Love and support are what they can give to each other, and they do so, without reserve or embarrassment. They are the ultimate in buddy systems.

A week after Matt's admission, the tube feeding is still not going well. Angela, 3B's head nurse, explains that Matthew is vomiting each night, bringing up all the formula, and usually the nasogastric tube as well. Kathy, the dietician, has tried every option — the formula has been diluted, the rate of flow decreased — but he is still not tolerating the feedings. Dr. Pritchard, naturally, is concerned. She consults with Dr. Gordon Pirie, who, in turn, orders special tests to determine the amount of oxygen in Matthew's blood while he is sleeping.

It is Friday, May 23. Don and I have been asked to meet with Sheila to discuss Matt's oxygen-level tests. She leads us to an office off the main ward and shuts the door behind us. Sheila is usually chirpy and cheerful but today she looks serious and concerned. She comes straight to the point.

"The problems with the tube-feeding are no longer a priority. I'm afraid Matthew couldn't be awakened this morning. He had taken a nap, and for at least fifteen minutes he couldn't be roused. Apparently, he's been falling asleep at inappropriate times for the past week. Everyone thought he was just tired, but it now appears more likely that his oxygen level is occasionally falling so low that he's blacking out — going unconscious.'' Sheila pauses briefly, then comes to the inevitable conclusion.

"I'm afraid that the disease is obviously progressing much faster than any of us anticipated."

There is silence in the office. As the reality sinks in, I recall the many times when we have found Matt asleep: often hunched over the hassock in front of the TV, repeatedly in the car, and his teacher, Mme. Smith, has even told me of his falling asleep during quiet time.

"We would like to know what you want us to do if Matthew stops breathing. Would you want him put on a respirator?"

A respirator? Oh God. . . Do we have to make the decision now? Why aren't we better prepared for this? We know how ill he is — the doctors have been telling us for months. But we thought we had more time.

I'm aware of one dominant feeling. It towers above the fears and sadness with which we're so well acquainted. Disappointment. Excruciating disappointment. Heart/lung transplants are new. The surgeons are still learning. Drugs are not perfected. Don and I had schemed together — "If we can just keep him going for another year or two, he'll have a better chance. The success rates will only improve." But now we learn there will be no waiting time. Matt will have to be a pioneer.

We discuss our son's life and impending death for the next ten minutes or so, until a final plan evolves. Sheila and Dr. Pirie will initiate inquiries regarding a transplant. As long as that is a reasonable possibility, we'll keep Matthew alive — on a respirator if necessary.

"In the meantime," Sheila continues, "we'll stop the night-feeds. The tests show that Matt's oxygen level while sleeping is only just high enough to keep him alive. Nighttime digestion is a luxury his body can't afford. We'll continue the tube-feeding during the day, between regular meals, while he is consciously breathing. Hopefully, this'll work better."

In the days ahead, food becomes an extreme nuisance for Matt. Everyone, from ourselves to the nurses to the cleaners, is telling him to "eat up." He doesn't want to "eat up" — he's not at all hungry. It becomes a game to avoid anyone who's planning to discuss his food intake. On more than one occasion, he shuts the door and props a chair against it, hoping to keep the dietician at bay! He soon finds, of course, that this doesn't work, and from then on, when his internal radar detects the approach of a threatening presence, he frequently and mysteriously disappears!

In addition to the lack of progress in his food intake, other complications arise, the worst of which is Matthew's attitude. He has been distinctly cool toward Don and me since his admission, but nothing as drastic as this.

"Why don't you go?" he says one day, soon after my arrival. His studied aloofness over the next few days becomes more and more pronounced. Pained, rejected, I browse in the children's library, talk to other parents, read the notice boards over and over again. And eat. How ironic. Matt is unable to eat, and I am unable to stop! Food has become a comforter, a friend. I take refuge in the cafeteria, devouring deep-fried shrimp by the plateful, and swilling them down with countless cups of sweet coffee. I dread returning to his room, to his cool manner, his averted eyes, and often a barb:

"Are you still here?" or "Haven't you gone yet?" I feel like a jilted lover — the unwanted girlfriend who has become an embarrassment, but won't give up.

"Why are you acting like this, Matthew?" I sometimes ask. He doesn't seem to know, and worse, doesn't seem to care. Kisses and hugs, once so willingly given, have become rare and precious gifts, grudgingly awarded. It's heartbreaking. I'm at my wit's end. Insulted if I stay, and feeling hurt and guilty if I leave, there's no winning. Don, too, receives the same treatment. He, however, reacts entirely differently: no whimpering, no hurt expressions, no searching for Freudian explanations. He's angry and lets Matthew know in no uncertain terms. It pays off — he fares much better than I, and gradually his doses of rejection become smaller and less concentrated.

Tony more than ever is Matt's friend and confidant, and his mother Katie has an invaluable role to play too. She becomes a substitute for me, filling in where I'm not allowed. I am totally excluded, a grovelling outsider. I can't help wondering what other parents think of me — this mother who comes to visit, and leaves within the hour. I try to tell them, casually, about Matt's attitude. I'm hoping that someone can relate to me. I desperately need to hear that Johnny or Susan "went through that." But they obviously didn't. No one seems to understand. Why would they? One day Matt is feeling especially tired. He climbs up onto Katie's knee and looks into her eyes.

"You're a very nice lady. I love you," he tells her.

"And I love you too, Matthew," she replies. In the midst of my pain, one positive feeling emerges. Relief — immense relief. Matt still has a mom of sorts.

The final crunch comes at the end of the month. It's Saturday, the last day of May. Matthew has been given a pass from the hospital and I'm planning to pick him up in the afternoon and take him to a family supper at the home of good friends, Paul and Jacqui Witt. Matthew knows the plan and has given it the nod.

The afternoon is warm and sunny, with a lazy weekend feel to it. The hospital underground parking lot is strangely quiet — many departments are closed on the weekend. The lobby, too, is deserted. Everything, it seems, is on hold — everything that is, except for illness itself. Matthew is sitting on his bed making paper airplanes.

"Hi, guy. How are you doing today?" I silently pray for a crumb of affection, and renewed ease in communication. Matt says nothing. There is no welcome, no acknowledgement. He focuses his attention firmly on his task, completely ignoring my presence.

"Are you ready to go?" I try another angle.

"Go where?"

"To Matthew and Jonathan's house. Remember, we're going for supper tonight."

There is no response. For the next twenty minutes we play a game of cat-and-mouse with words and emotions. His message is clear and hurtful. He is not going to leave the hospital today. He would rather be here than at home.

"Why don't you just go?" he demands.

I cannot give up that easily. Quelling tears and nursing the lowest self-esteem in the history of motherhood, I propose taking him downstairs for a ride in his wheelchair. That's always a winner — after all, the shop may be open with its splendid array of candy, books and toys.

"We've got to talk about this, Matthew," I tell him as the elevator discharges us into the almost deserted lobby.

"I'm sorry that you're ill, but it's not my fault. I love you and want to be with you so I can help, but your attitude to me is both unkind and rude. Have I done something to upset you?"

"No."

"Have I said something you don't like?"

"No."

We amble down the empty corridor toward the clinic areas. Matt is hunched forward in his familiar position, straining to utilize every part of his lungs. I feel desperate and am fast running out of reserve.

"Do you blame me that you're ill?"

"No."

We have retraced our route and have reached the lobby again. I can stand no more. Sitting quickly, I turn his chair around so that we are facing each other, eyeball to eyeball.

"Then what is it? Why are you doing this? You're hurting me, Matthew. You're hurting me."

He is taken aback by the sudden outburst, but only a little.

"I'm sorry. I can't help it," he replies, dispassionately. And, in spite of my anguish, something tells me he's speaking the truth. He can't help it. It's as though he has been programmed — maybe under the heading of "coping". His subconscious mind is calling the shots.

There's no more to say. Back on 3B, beaten and sick at heart, I say goodbye. There is no response. The brown head is bowed, already intent on the details of the paper airplane.

I am, without doubt, an impaired driver on this sunny Saturday afternoon. I sob hysterically all the way down Oak Street, and then, with city traffic left behind, vent my anger at the God who seems to have deserted us.

"Where are you, God?" I yell in mocking tones. "Isn't it enough that Matthew's so ill? But this too? What do you think you're doing? Are you on holiday? Long coffee-break, maybe? It's disgusting. That's what it is. Disgusting."

But at this moment, God, like Matthew, offers no response.

Dr. Le Page shows me into his small office on the ground floor. A tall, attractive man, he is fascinated by the trappings of the human mind, and anxious to resolve its numerous conflicts. I had phoned Sheila first thing on Monday morning to tell her that we urgently needed help. And help had arrived quickly. Dr. Le Page, a hospital psychologist, had been consulted, and had spent some time with Matthew. I can hardly wait for the answers, and, even more, some advice. Dr. Le Page talks rapidly, describing the many possible factors which are certainly influencing our son's behaviour.

"The first is somewhat basic," he says. "Matthew has lost control in nearly every area of his life. He's lost control over the state of his health, his body, over his options to be at home or in a hospital, over normal physical activities — bike rides and ball games — that he used to love. He has no say in what happens to his body here at the hospital: blood is taken, stomach tubes inserted, thoracenteses performed, medication given — there is no choice." He pauses briefly. "You are the one area where he does have some control. He can choose and dictate, to a certain extent, whether you are with him or not. He knows that you love him unconditionally, which makes you what we call a safe target. It is not meant unkindly, and it is definitely not rational. But it does give him some measure of control."

I nod, acknowledging some comprehension of what he is telling me. I am immensely relieved. At least there is an explanation.

Dr. Le Page continues: "Children with catastrophic illness frequently mature to well above their age level, and Matthew is no exception. Although he's not yet seven, he has actually matured to the level of a nine- or ten-year-old in some respects. He probably well understands the significance of his illness at that age level, but has not developed comparable coping abilities. He cannot verbalize his feelings well at this age and stage, so his anger and frustrations must find other outlets. Again, you are a safe target.

"Another possibility is that he may blame you, in a highly irrational manner, for the fact that he is ill. You are, after all, his mother, who should nurture and protect him, and it may seem to Matthew that you are falling down on the job."

"I can certainly relate to that," I interrupt. "Even I feel that way sometimes, in spite of it being irrational. I often feel guilty that we've failed to protect him. It makes me mad, too. We've always been so careful — a helmet when he's on his bike, a lifejacket around water, never allowed him on the road — you name it, we did it! It seems so unfair."

Tony Le Page nods sympathetically. In his line of work he has plenty of opportunity to observe the unfairness of life.

"And there's more," he continues. "He knows that you love and accept him when he's well and normal. But what about now? He may be wondering if you still love him now that he's ill and handicapped."

What a harrying possibility! How unthinkable! I struggle momentarily with the need to rush back to 3B and reassure Matthew that nothing has changed in our feelings for him. This interview, however, is too important to interrupt with emotional outbursts.

"So you see, there are many possibilities to explain Matthew's hurtful behaviour. And there's one that I haven't mentioned yet, which is probably the most significant." Pausing, he chooses his words with care.

"Matthew may be trying to protect, not just himself, but you too. By distancing himself from you, both physically and emotionally, he may be hoping to lessen the pain of separation, which his illness is likely to bring. This is all on the subconscious level, of course." It doesn't seem possible. A six-year-old trying to prepare for his own death! What's more, trying to prepare us, too!

"So what can I do, Dr. Le Page? How do I deal with it?"

There is no hesitation.

"Stay with him," he advises. "If he suggests that you leave, simply tell him that you love him and would prefer to stay. Let him know you'll be sitting in his room, and if he wants to be with you, that's great, and if he doesn't, that's all right too. But make it clear that you choose to be close by anyway. And here's one more thing I should mention. If you can be with him late in the evening, when the bustle of the day is over and the floor is settling for the night, you'll have a much better chance of him talking to you. Really talking — about things that matter.'' I rise to go.

"Thank you, Dr. Le Page. We'll give it a try. Things can't get any worse, that's for sure.''

It feels good to have a plan and some guidelines again. Like most parents with seriously ill children, we're anxious to do our best. We don't need regrets too. I leave the tiny office full of hope.

The next day, armed with my new ammunition, I arrive at Children's Hospital by two o'clock. Matt is sitting cross-legged on the bed playing with his Transformers. He looks up briefly as I enter, then continues with his game.

"Hi, guy!'' I start cheerfully. "How are you today?'' There is no response, of course. None was expected. "I've brought some clean pyjamas for you. I'll put them in your cupboard. I've also brought a jar of peaches and some cereal. I'll just leave them here by your bed, and you can help yourself.'' Nothing.

"It would be nice if you'd say thank you when people do things for you, Matthew.''

A mumbled response passes, just barely, as a reluctant thank you.

I take a magazine from my bag, and settle into an easy chair. I know I won't have long to wait.

"What are you here for? You don't need to stay.'' I take a deep breath. My lines are well rehearsed.

"I know I don't, Matt. I could go home anytime. However, I want to stay close by. You don't have to be with me if you don't want to, but I am choosing to stay with you.'' There is silence. Matt returns to the Transformers, and I to my magazine. After a few minutes, he slides off the bed and leaves the room. He returns after half an hour.

"Are you still here?'' he demands. "Why don't you go home?'' His voice is cold and unfriendly.

"I don't want to go home, Matt. I like being close to you. I'm just going to sit here and read.'' Again, he doesn't stay for long — and repeats his brief demands on returning for his supper tray. The evening, however, is blissfully free of confrontations, and by the time I leave for the night, I know I have a foot in the door.

The next day, Matt makes his chilling demands again, but only once. Is it wishful thinking, or do I detect a hint of relief when I insist on staying? It feels so good. I am in the driver's seat once more.

Day Three. "Hey Mom, when can we go to Expo?'' I kiss him on his head, risking rejection again. He wraps his thin arms around my neck, and rests his cheek against mine.

A few days later, he shyly hands me a small blue card. On the front is a cute dog with big, fluffy ears and a heart on its chest. Inside is written:

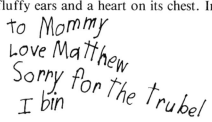

Expo. There has been talk of little else for the past two years. Now it's in full swing, and Expo '86 is everything that was promised and more. It is a wonderful, sensational party put on by people of many nations. The whole world has been invited — and apparently accepted! Vancouverites are hosts and guests all at the same time. It is first-rate entertainment and fabulous technology. It's a feast of sights, sounds and moods. It's a celebration of life itself.

"Matthew wants to know if he can go on the Scream Machine, Dr. Pirie. What do you think?" I am of course passing the buck, but don't always want to be the one to say no. The Scream Machine — the ultimate rollercoaster — knocks the wind out of the average person. Matthew has none to spare. Dr. Pirie's response is predictable.

"Aw, not fair, Mom," Matt protests. He soon discovers, however, that there is much more to Expo than the thrills of the Scream Machine.

The sunny afternoon is perfect for our intended outing. Don and I pick Elizabeth up from school promptly at three, then drive to Children's Hospital. Matthew is ready and waiting, and excited. Borrowing a hospital wheelchair, we sign the necessary release form, and, promising to have a great time, head for the Expo site.

Balloons and flags, clowns and cotton candy, breathtaking colour and excited children, fascinating exhibits, constant movement, crowded trains and skyrides, long queues, sensational films, exotic aromas — Expo is all these and much, much more.

There are benefits, we find, to having an invalid in our midst. Instead of lining up, like thousands of others, for the skytrain, we are ushered to the exit ramp for priority treatment. There are special arrangements for wheelchairs at many of the pavilions, and on the skyrides, too.

Like us, the children are mesmerized by the magnitude and calibre of such an enormous exhibition. One of the highlights of the evening is a visit to the Telecom Canada Pavilion. The circular theatre with its spectacular 360-

degree film of Canada is exceptional, and the children enjoy the display in the adjoining hall. Matthew, in particular, loves the talking phones on which he can speak to his favourite Disney characters. A good friend, Valerie Ward, is a hostess in the pavilion, so we enjoy some V.I.P. treatment.

And then, inevitably, the Scream Machine.

"Be sure to hold on tight, Elizabeth. Don, you check the safety bar. Have you emptied your pockets? Keep your hands in, won't you? Matthew and I will be here." Don and Elizabeth exchange knowing glances at my fussing, and hurry away to join the line-up. Matt and I watch in silence as the car climbs slowly up the steep hill. The ride is aptly named — some of its victims are screaming even before the first descent. A chorus of shrieks attends the plummeting cars, and by the time they reach the sharp curves and awesome loops, a crescendo of protest and delight can be heard across the fair site. After their ride, Don and Elizabeth look mighty pleased with themselves.

"I kept my eyes open the whole time. There's nothing to it." Elizabeth can scarcely wait to go again. Matt, hunched over in his wheelchair, says nothing.

A few minutes later, passing the beautiful baroque carousel, Matt asks if he can have a ride. Elizabeth would like to join him, and is peeved at being denied. But it is Matt's turn — and he alone will be allowed on this one. An attendant helps him onto a magnificent horse, and the music, enchanting and haunting, begins to play. The small, pale boy, in a world of his own, moves with it, round and round, up and down. Time pauses. A memory is created — one that will last forever.

It's early evening and I'm pushing Matthew's wheelchair. We cross the lobby and head down the corridors toward the hospital cafeteria. Matt is playing with a favourite Transformer. He is deep in thought.

"Mom," he says.

"Yes, dear?"

"Will there be Transformers in heaven?"

My mouth is dry and my stomach suddenly in knots.

"I don't know for sure, but heaven is full of wonderful things, so maybe there'll be Transformers too."

The moment passes. The subject changes.

A few nights later, I am tucking him into bed. The night nurses are turning out lights, giving medications, and switching off the TV sets.

"Mom."

"Yes, hon?"

"What's the most important part of the body?"

I remember Tony Le Page's words: ". . . a much better chance of him talking to you. Really talking — about things that matter."

"Well, let's see," I stall. "The brain is very important, and the heart."

I'm plucking up courage to suggest the lungs, when he jumps right in. He's three steps ahead of me.

"And the spirit. The spirit is important too." It is not so much a question as a statement.

"Yes, hon, but I don't think of the spirit as part of the body because the spirit lives on when the body dies."

He nods in acknowledgement, says his prayers and falls asleep.

"Goodnight, dear Matthew. God bless."

Chapter Nine

Heart/lung transplants are new to the world of medicine, and consequently, there are few hospitals in the world where they are performed. Drs. Pirie, Adderley and Le Blanc start checking out the possibilities and making inquiries. There is one Canadian hospital on the list, University Hospital in London, Ontario. Unfortunately, they have not yet started paediatric heart/lung transplants.

So the search turns toward the States and England. Stanford, Boston, Pittsburgh and Minneapolis are the main centres in the States, and Harefield Hospital, near London, is the primary choice in England.

Several days later, when I arrive back from supper, Dr. Pirie is waiting outside Matt's room. We talk of Expo, of the excitement in the city, of the upcoming "Childrun." I feign a calmness I do not feel, sensing he has some news. Finally, he tells me, as gently as he can,

"Dr. Adderley heard back from Stanford today. I'm afraid they can't take Matthew. . ."

Half an hour later, Don arrives on the floor. We wander out to the roof, to the freedom of the evening air.

"What reason did they give?" he asks, recovering from the first sharp pains of disappointment.

"They say he's too high-risk. Because of the chest surgery and infections, there'll be scarring and adhesions. Apparently it makes it much more complicated."

"Complicated isn't impossible" he says, not without bitterness.

"I guess they can't give everyone a chance, Don. There aren't enough organs to go around. They have to select only the best bets, the people most likely to make it."

"So what now?" he asks. "Do we just give up? With a fighter like Matt, do we not even try?"

The question is lost in the wail of a siren. Below us on Oak Street, the traffic slows, coming to a reverent crawl. The screaming ambulance weaves a route, cautiously defies the lights, then speeds towards the Emergency entrance.

"We'll just have to wait and see," I answer. "We haven't heard back from the other centres. Hopefully someone else will take him. It's the only chance we have.''

Matt is discharged from hospital and we go home to wait. He has added a few pounds to his thin frame, and we are equipped with supplies for tube-feeding, should he backslide on his intake of regular food. He goes straight back to school. It's nearly the end of term, and an opportunity to see his teacher and friends and join in the inevitable outings and festivities. On good days, I fear we are moving too fast in our search for a transplant.

''He looks so well,'' friends tell me, and I can't help but agree. Is it possible that the doctors are wrong? On bad days, our doubts disappear, replaced by the gnawing fear that we are rapidly running out of time.

Friday, June 20. The children are both at school. Don's in his study, paying bills and sorting out paperwork. I'm clearing the breakfast table, feeding the dog, doing laundry — Mrs. Average Housewife on a Friday morning. The phone rings and Don answers it. Something in his tone draws me to the doorway of his study. Seeing me, he beckons urgently.

''When can we leave, Dr. Pirie?'' he asks, making notes on a pad as he listens.

''Katie has family in England, of course.'' He pauses while Dr. Pirie supplies more information.

England!

My knees turn to jelly. Sinking onto the carpet, I prop myself against the wall.

''We'll talk to you soon. And thank you, Dr. Pirie. Thank you very much.'' Don replaces the phone and turns to face me. His voice is anything but steady.

''That was Dr. Pirie. Mr. Murad from Harefield will see Matthew, if we can get him over there.''

It's wonderful news. It's a chance for Matthew. It's also terrifying.

Silence hangs heavy between us. It's several minutes before either of us speaks. This is it — decision time. No longer can we ignore the nagging doubts and fears which we've been so carefully avoiding.

''He looks so well at the moment. Are you sure we're not rushing too fast?'' I ask.

''Don't forget, he's been blacking out — and for some time now. Besides, the prednisone makes him look better than he is.'' I nod in reluctant agreement.

''Remember what Dr. Pirie said, about some things being worse than death? What if something goes wrong? What if he ends up paralysed or brain-damaged? What if he suffers? He's been through so much already. I can't bear for him to suffer any more.''

Don speaks slowly. He has obviously thought this through.

"We don't have a crystal ball. But all being well, he won't suffer before the surgery. The operation itself is probably the crucial part. If he dies on the table, he won't have suffered unduly. If he survives the surgery, any subsequent suffering, while he recovers, will be justified."

We juggle the possibilities, weighing one against the other. There are risks, uncertainties and question marks at every turn. In the final analysis, only one thing is clear. Without the transplant, Matthew will die. With it, he may live. There is no more to be said.

The rest of Friday is spent in telling family and friends the exciting news. In the evening, Don alone breaks it to the children. His presentation is distinctly upbeat: ". . .a great chance. . . a wonderful opportunity. . . a new, healthy set of lungs . . ."

Matt says nothing, but appears to be relieved. Elizabeth pouts.

"Why can't I come too, Daddy?" She chews nervously on strands of her long blond hair.

"You won't have any fun, Beth," he explains. "We'll be sitting around in waiting rooms for hours on end. There'll be no time for outings. You'll be bored silly."

"I can take some books and read. I love reading. And I can watch TV. Maybe I could stay with Granny Petal." Her blue eyes are brighter than usual.

"No, Beth," Don replies firmly. "Granny lives two hundred miles from the hospital. Let's keep things simple. Auntie Lonnie would love to have you, and you'll have a great time. Why, between swimming in the pool and going to the malls, you'll be spoiled rotten! Di's invited you to Kamloops too. You'll love that, won't you?" The truth is, we'll have no time for Elizabeth. No time — and probably no energy. There really is no choice.

That night Don and I discuss the events of the day. At my insistence, he relates the talk with Beth and Matthew. "You did mention the heart, too, didn't you?" I ask him. His depiction of "putting the rotten, old, diseased lungs in the garbage" and "replacing them with brand-new ones" is laudable, but there is no mention of the heart. He looks a little uncomfortable.

"Well no," he says sheepishly. I thought it might be better to start with the lungs until he gets used to the idea. Besides, the heart is different somehow."

"He'll have to know," I shrug. He's going to hear "heart/lung transplant" bandied about soon enough; we don't want him to think we're not being straight with him. Don agrees. The omission must be rectified as soon as possible. I lie awake for a long time trying to choose just the right words.

The following morning, Saturday, Matt is sitting colouring in the living room. I wander in nonchalantly, and perch on the sofa.

"What are you colouring, Matt?"

"Optimus Prime," without looking up.

"That's your favourite, isn't it?" He nods, intent on the job.

"Oh, by the way, fella, you know Daddy was telling you about your sick lungs being replaced by new ones?" The artist grunts in acknowledgement. "Well, he forgot to mention that you get a new heart too. It all works as one unit, you see — the old heart and lungs come out together, and the new heart and lungs go in together." I pause for breath, bracing myself for the inevitable questions.

"OK," he says. "What are we doing today, Mom?"

That evening a close friend comes around for supper. Joan is the principal of an elementary school in Burnaby. Today is the first day of their summer recess. She's tired and stressed, and looking forward to the break. She is also elated. She and Alistair have been trying to adopt a child from Peru, and have recently been successful. A baby girl called Laura is waiting for them in Lima. They plan to fly down next week, and bureaucracy willing, return with their daughter by the end of the summer.

"So, tell me what's happening," she demands, greetings perfunctorily dispensed with. "Here, I'll mash the potatoes." She listens intently as I describe yesterday's important phone call.

"That's great! So when do you leave?"

"That's a good question. The problem is. . . help yourself to the nibbles. . . that Matt can't fly, at least not in a regular aircraft. Do you remember that awful flight coming back from the Mayo? Well, his lungs are worse now. The last pulmonary function test indicated that less than thirty percent of his lungs are working. He simply wouldn't survive in the rarefied atmosphere of a commercial airliner."

"But couldn't you give him oxygen? Here, let me stir the gravy. That worked on the last flight, didn't it?"

"No, that's another problem. Matthew's disease has progressed to the point where giving him oxygen only makes matters worse. His breathing depends on a low oxygen level as opposed to a high carbon dioxide level. It's known as 'Catch 22'."

"Well, you know what you need, then?" she says, picking at the crispiest chicken skin. "You need a private plane. Do you know anyone who's got one?"

"Oh sure, Joanie. Don, where's our list of friends who have their own planes?"

"No, I'm serious, you guys. Mmm . . . roast potatoes! Can I just pinch that little one? You'd be surprised how many businessmen, right here in Vancouver, own private jets," Joanie reels off several well-known names, without even having to think.

"I'll bet Mitch knows some of them," she says, referring to a mutual friend. "And Joanne Stan. Do you remember her from university days? This chicken's delicious. . . well, if there's plenty. . . are you sure you don't want that skin, Don?"

"Joanie, we can't just ask someone to lend us their plane for the weekend," I protest weakly.

"Why not? You're in a desperate situation. It calls for desperate measures. People like to help, if given the chance. Is that rhubarb pie? Yes, please. Oh, don't whip the cream just for me — I love it either way."

Once supper is finished, Joan starts making phone calls. The first is to our mutual friend, Mitch Taylor. As one of the movers and shakers in Vancouver's business circles, Mitch's contacts are considerable. Joan talks for several minutes, then replaces the phone.

"He's going to check around and see what he can do," she says, thumbing once more through the big directory.

"Joanne? It's Joan. Listen, we need some help." Joanne phones her fiance, Keith Morgan, who calls moments later to talk to Joan. The same details are outlined again.

"My old friend J. Bob Carter has his own plane, of course," Keith tells Joanie, "but he's out of the country at present. I'll try and track him down though." And then, "I'm a reporter with *The Province*, you know. I wonder if I could talk to one of your friends. I'd be interested in doing a story — it could be helpful for them too."

We're most reluctant. Life is tough enough, thank you, without the added stress that publicity could bring. But we're asking for help, and feel we can't say no. I'm far from happy as I take the phone. The English-accented voice is neither pushy nor threatening. Keith assures me that he will handle the story personally — it won't be sensationalized.

"Publicity may help in unexpected ways," he says. "Don will be away 'til Monday night, you say. I'll come round on Tuesday morning then. And we'll start working on the plane right now."

An hour later, with promises to keep close tabs on developments, Joanie leaves for home. "I don't know why you keep inviting me, when all I do is eat your food," she quips, before disappearing into the night.

The next day at morning service, our minister, Dale Cuming, announces that we are taking Matthew to England for a transplant, and that a fund has been set up to help with our expenses. This comes as no surprise to us as, upon our return from the Mayo Clinic in May, Dale had mentioned that a number of people had suggested a fund to help with our medical costs. We had gratefully declined at the time, because the provincial Medical Services Plan would cover much of our bill and we were able to absorb the remainder.

"However," Don had joked, "we won't turn you down if we need to go for a transplant!" The church had quietly gone ahead, organizing everything in anticipation. All that was needed was our OK.

Another friend has plans to help us too. Russ Stogryn, himself a surgeon, has monitored Matthew's illness in his own personal way right from the beginning. He has always been there, an unobtrusive strength in the background — the overseer, keeping check at a distance.

"It's time I talked to the B.C. Lions' Society," he says, when Don calls to fill him in on the latest developments. "This is exactly the kind of thing they support. I've looked into it a bit already. The head man is a Mr. Townsend; I'll call him right away."

The receiver is no sooner replaced than the phone rings again, jangling loudly. Don answers, as usual, and I can quickly tell from his tone that whatever the news, it's most welcome. The call over, he turns and hugs me tightly. Tears well in his eyes, threatening to spill down his cheeks.

"That was Dr. Pirie," he says. "An I.C.U. doctor is going to be flying with us. We won't be on our own. His name is Macnab, Andrew Macnab. He's apparently head of the air ambulance team. He'll be taking care of Matthew. . . we won't be on our own."

I wrap my arms around Don's neck and lay my head against his chest. Slowly, very slowly, we sway together, rocking gently from side to side. The sun's warm rays stream through the window, melting taut muscles, caressing our souls. We dance for what seems like a long, long time, moving as one to the soundless music.

Don has a momentous decision to make. Should he carry on fishing — the salmon runs this year are predicted to be exceptional — maybe catching up with Matthew and me in England in a few weeks' time, or should he forget it for this season, tie up the boat and cut his losses? He carefully weighs what facts we have, but most of these are purely conditional — there are too many uncertainties. In the final analysis, there can be only one decision. "There'll be more salmon to catch next year," he says. "I've only got one son." He leaves on Sunday morning to bring his boat from Ucluelet, on the rugged west coast, to the bigger marina at Port Alberni.

Later that afternoon, our friends the Dregers — Di, Glenn, and Glenn's sister-in-law, Carol — arrive from Kamloops. With Di and Glenn's children, Heidi and Jason, they've driven the four-hour journey to see Matthew and say goodbye. Carol has brought diaries for each of us. "You may want to keep notes," she tells us. "You'll probably have days when it will help to write things down."

They can only stay for an hour before having to leave for home, but when they do, it's with an extra passenger. Thor, wedged between Glenn and Di and looking utterly confused, has found a good home for the summer.

The next day I phone Andrew Macnab, just to make contact. "We're so relieved that you're coming too," I tell him. Andrew, it seems, has already been at work.

"I've started checking on flights to England. The main airlines only fly at night, and as you know, Matthew's condition worsens when he's asleep. Not only that, the commercial flights are pressurized to 8,000 feet — that's not enough oxygen for Matthew. I'm afraid it's not looking too good."

The following days are a whirlwind of increasing momentum. The phone rings incessantly.

"I'm still trying to locate Mr. Townsend," Russ says. "There was a big Lions event in town this weekend. It's hard to track him down. Anyway, I'll keep trying. Talk to you soon."

"You'll need some clothes for England, Katie," Geraldine suggests. "When are you free? We could choose some together. What size are you? I'll ask the lady at Sharelle's to pick some out, to save you time. How about tomorrow?"

Keith Morgan phones. "J. Bob Carter is in the Philippines, but there's been a hurricane and the lines are all down. I've left a message with his office. I'm sure he'll check in as soon as he can. I'll be round as planned on Tuesday morning."

My sister Joan calls from England. "I've spoken to a Mrs. King, who boards outpatients at Harefield. She's keeping accommodation for you. Phone back when you know your schedule."

"Just a minute of your time." It's Margi. "People are asking me what they can do. They want to help but don't know how. Let's just take a minute and make a list . . ."

Joy: "I've made some muffins; I'll just pop them down. Stephi said a little prayer for Matthew at lunchtime. We're all praying, you know . . ."

Another friend, Giselle: "If Elizabeth would like to come to French camp with us, Michelle would love the company. Just let us know."

And my dear friend Sandy. Every day. "Now, anything at all, Kathleen. You know I'm just a minute away."

Geraldine again: "I've taken the liberty of making a hair appointment for you on Thursday. Exotic Trends at eleven o'clock. Would you mind confirming with them? The bill is taken care of by the way."

Dale Cuming calls. "We have a friend who's looking for a place to stay this summer. He'd happily house-sit for you."

And then, Dr. Pirie, with a sobering, frightening reminder: "You do understand that Mr. Murad has made no promises? Matthew will have to be assessed." Don replaces the phone slowly. "What if we get all the way over there, and he can't do it?" he groans. "How would we ever get him back on our own?" The prospect is overwhelming.

Keith Morgan arrives punctually on Tuesday morning. I guess him to be somewhere in his mid-thirties — a few years younger than us anyway. He's outgoing and congenial — a personality well suited to his job. We start at the beginning and relate the story of Matthew's illness. He's painstaking over the details and fascinated by the possibilities now offered by medical technology. He leaves shortly before lunch, telling us that a photographer will arrive after three to take pictures of Matt. In spite of all Keith's reassurances, we feel very stressed. It's scary to "go public."

At 3:15 a *Province* photographer, Colin Savage, arrives at the door. Matthew has gone after school to play with his pal Gregory. I jump in the van and rush to Sandy's house. I quickly explain the situation to them. "Aw, Mom, we're right in the middle of a game," Matt protests. Talk about the reluctant star.

"Come on, fella. It'll just take a few minutes, and I'll bring you straight back to Greg's house, OK?" He thinks about this for a moment before agreeing. "All right, Mom. But only for a few minutes." The session, does in fact, last for an hour. But Colin makes it into a game. It's fun for both the children. And the resulting pictures justify every second.

The next morning, Wednesday, June 25, page three of *The Province* carries a big colour picture of Matthew. He's sitting cross-legged on the lawn, playing with Optimus Prime. The caption, in large, thick, print, comes straight to the point. "URGENT! PLANE NEEDED FOR BOY." The photo is excellent, and Keith, as promised, has handled the story with impeccable taste. The phone starts ringing, and the doorbell, too. Friends and neighbours call to offer support of every kind.

We have all heard of "the power of the press." It's an expression often used in a negative context. For us it is extremely positive — a catalyst far beyond our wildest dreams.

Midmorning. Don answers the phone for the umpteenth time. It's

Martti Huttunen, an acquaintance and neighbour. He had read the *Province* story, he tells Don, and immediately contacted a business associate in Alberta. John Zigarlick, president of Echo Bay Mines, in Alberta, has offered a Lear jet complete with crew for our journey. There will be no charge.

We all receive gifts in our lives — big ones, small ones, sentimental or official ones. This gift, with its forty-thousand-dollar price tag, from someone who doesn't even know us, falls into no ordinary category. We are deeply moved.

Incredibly, before the day is out, there will be two other offers of planes, one from Wardair and the other from J. Bob Carter, who has finally escaped from the storm-ravaged Philippines and arrived safely in Tokyo.

Suddenly, everything begins to fall into place. Don contacts B.C. Med and learns, to our enormous relief, that they will pay the medical bills. Because a heart/lung transplant isn't available for Matthew here, they will pick up the tab in other countries, but only up to the estimated Canadian cost. Had we been going to the States, we would have had to pay thousands of dollars in surplus charges. With England's relatively lower scale, Matt will be completely covered.

Russ calls. He has contacted Mr. Townsend and the news is great. The Lions have offered to pay our bills for board and lodging — and anything else that B.C. Med doesn't cover. Can you imagine? At one point we had discussed selling everything we owned, if that's what it came to.

I have errands to do in town. Leaving Don to answer the phone, I hurry down to our local Royal Bank. Much to my amazement, Matthew's picture is taped on the door. Another one is posted inside, along with the *Province* story. The bank, too, is starting a fund to help us.

"TV? Oh no, Don. I really can't face it!" I've raced home to tell him about the Royal Bank fund. Before I can get it out, I'm hearing that Channel 13 is sending a news team out within the hour. I'm not thrilled.

"Now calm down. It'll be all right. Look how we were over the newspaper — and it was fine. It was more than fine."

At lunchtime, Rick Hoogendoorn arrives with a cameraman in tow. Rick is a concerned, soft-spoken man, probably in his early twenties. He has an air of not wishing to intrude. We confirm the story in the *Province* and tell him about the offer of a plane. He takes notes as we talk — gentle, unobtrusive, non-threatening. By the time he gets around to asking if they could have some film of Matthew, my fears are dispelled.

"He's in school," I tell him. "I'll go and see if he'll come home through lunch break. I won't be long."

Cliff Drive Elementary is only a mile away, and within five minutes, I have reached Matthew's classroom. Recess has just begun, and the room is still full of children. At that very moment, an older boy, possibly in grade three or four, enters with the *Province* clipping. He's obviously a showman. He holds the picture up for all the children to see and someone starts to cheer. Matt is standing by his desk; from his smile and flushed face, I can see he's enjoying the attention. The cheers fade away and Mr. Showbiz takes his place on centre stage again. To my horror, he starts to read the story aloud. Amazingly, no one but me appears to flinch at "terminally ill" and "last hope." Maybe the children don't understand. Or maybe, like Matthew, they're able to block out the unacceptable. The boy finishes reading, and exits with a flourish. The children start drifting off, lured by hunger and playmates.

"Hi, Matthew," I start. He hardly notices my presence. Brittany, a pretty, blond, blue-eyed first-grader is standing with him. She smiles up at me, polite and charming.

"I'm going to stay with Matthew for recess," she announces. "I'm not going to leave him." They smile shyly at each other, and I know instinctively that Rick Hoogendoorn is out of luck. I try my best: ". . . TV. . . cameraman. . . news tonight. . . back to school later. . ." Brittany's conquest is absolute. Matthew is going nowhere!

Rick and his cameraman return at three, and the item is aired on the news at five-thirty. It is tasteful and accurate, leaving us with no regrets.

Someone has left a present on the doorstep. "Dear Matthew," reads the unsigned card, "We're All Wanting You To Get Well Soon." Inside the unwrapped box is a large, soft lion. His smile is shy and unassuming. He sports a big red heart on his chest. His name, in large letters, is proudly and pointedly displayed — LIONHEART.

Somewhere in the dark distance, a telephone rings. I pull the sheet over my head. Don bats blindly at the wall. "Hello," he says, finally, his voice weary with sleep. I re-emerge to check the time. Five after six! Who on earth could be calling at this hour!

"He's still asleep, Matthew. It's only six o'clock. You'll see him at school today." Don replaces the phone and groans.

"That was Matthew B. wanting to say goodbye. Can you believe it? At this hour?"

"I think that's sweet." I yawn, and am immediately asleep once more.

It is, in fact, just the beginning of a deluge of phone calls, and a fitting start to Thursday, June 26. The next call comes at eight o'clock, and the phone rings constantly all through the day. Geraldine, with her usual E.S.P., brings over an answering machine — it's the only way we can get anything done.

I race down to school at 10 a.m. to take in part of the closing assembly. The principal, grandfatherly Mr. Riley, is retiring this year, and a special farewell has been planned in his honour. He smiles and blushes at the well-deserved accolades. At one point, he makes reference to Cliff Drive's fund for Matthew — news, indeed, to me. "I'm sure we all want to wish Matthew well in England," he ends.

Elizabeth and Matthew go back to Geraldine's to play with Andrea and Robert, while I get pampered at Exotic Trends. When I get home, Don is chatting intently with Keith Morgan.

Another phone call. It's Andrew Macnab.

"Just wanting to fill you in on some of the details," he says. "One of the respiratory technologists, Jeff Vachon, will be travelling with us too. We're planning to use some very new equipment to monitor Matthew's oxygen levels."

Both the medics, it seems, are delighted with the jet.

"The Lear 35 can pressurize to 1000 feet when it's flying at 28,000," Andrew tells Don.

"Matthew's condition demands that we have a low altitude flight with the cabin pressure maintained as close to sea level as possible."

Andrew goes on to explain that depending on the monitor readings, the medics and pilots will determine together how low or high the plane must fly in order to keep Matt oxygenated.

"As you probably know," he adds, "we need to fly as high as possible for speed and fuel efficiency, but needless to say, Matthew's health comes first."

"When are we leaving, Andrew?" Don asks.

"Tomorrow morning, all being well — and definitely no later than nine. Matthew can run into problems when sleeping. We're wanting to travel only within his daytime."

A phone call from Russ. He's now our liaison not only with the B.C. Lions' Society, but also with Children's Hospital and the company donating the plane.

"There's a minor problem with insurance for the medics," he tells us. "I'll get back to you shortly."

I call Joan in Putney.

"We should be arriving at Gatwick on Saturday morning, your time. We'll phone when we know for sure."

The children are home from school.

"Probably tomorrow," we tell them, with no time to worry about their feelings.

Katie, Tony and Marcus Di Iuorio arrive.

"Tony insisted on coming. I know you must be busy, but we had to come and see him. You don't mind, do you?" Tony has stooped and is giving Matt a bearhug.

"We're so glad you did. Welcome to the zoo . . ."

Our community cable TV station: "We can't find an interviewer. Do you think you could ask each other questions?"

Another friend and well-wisher arrives at the door. "I thought you could probably use a few muffins. . ."

Sandy and Greg are here, bearing presents for the children. "Now, Kathleen, we've come to help. What can we do?"

The phone again. "We've found someone. He hasn't done much interviewing, though. Could they come over right away?"

They arrive within minutes. The interviewer, John, is a likable man, probably a little older than ourselves. Don, Elizabeth, Matt and I sit on the brick fireplace, down in the rec room. Our friends stand around the room watching, mainly in amusement. The camera light is on. "Take one," the man calls.

"Good evening. We're at the home of Dan and Katie Ekroth . . ." Both children start laughing.

"It's Don," Matt tells him.

"Take two," the man calls.

This time Don has problems. The right words won't surface.

"Take three."

"Good evening. We're at the home of Don and Kathy Ekroth."

"It's Katie!" the children yell together, rolling around in hysterics. Our friends laugh with them.

"Take four."

At last! This one goes well. The interview is almost over.

"And do you have anything you want to add, Matthew?" John asks. Matt looks straight into the camera. He is serious now. "I just want to thank the people," he says, "to thank them for everything."

Katie, Tony and Marcus have to leave. Tony lingers, hugging his friend for a last time.

"See you when you get back, pal," he says, tears glistening in his eyes.

Friends arrive bearing supper, just as they did yesterday. Geraldine and her husband, Laurie, come back for the evening.

"We'll tidy up and answer the phone," says Geraldine. "You still have to pack."

Another phone call, this time from Winnipeg, 1500 miles away.

"You don't know me; I saw Matthew's story in the paper. We've been to Harefield, too. Our daughter, Mary, was under Mr. Murad's care. I thought it might be helpful to fill you in on some details. . ." As it turns out, Susan Shallcross is more than helpful. She prepares us well for Harefield. We are left greatly encouraged, but with no illusions.

Russ and Shirley arrive, and Sandy's husband, Ken. Somebody helps me pack. Still others clean the house. Someone else takes care of the phone.

Sandy puts the children to bed.

"Goodnight sweetheart," she says to Elizabeth, stooping to plant a kiss on her cheek. "We'll see you in the morning. Sleep well."

Matt is almost ready too. Sandy sits on the side of his bed and helps him up onto her knee. They talk of the exciting trip ahead, of the many neat times they've spent together, of how soon he'll be back home again. And they make their plans for the future, dreaming of brighter tomorrows.

"The waterslides for sure," he says. "That'll be the first thing!"

Sandy gives him a big hug and kisses him goodnight.

"We all love you, Matthew," she says as she props him up on his pillows. She stays until he seems to have settled, then quietly tiptoes from the room.

At ten o'clock, Russ is still working on the insurance details. He sits in his car in the driveway talking into his cellular phone, which has almost become an extension of his ear. At ten-thirty, he appears in the hall, beaming.

By midnight, our friends have all left. The rooms are clean, our bags are packed.

There is a knock on the door. "Here's milk for the morning," says Russ, holding up a carton. "Sleep well."

Friday, June 27, 6:30 a.m. The alarm by our bed rings loudly and Don swats at it as usual, grappling for control. I've been up for more than an hour now, stimulated by fear, excitement, and awareness of unfinished tasks. Watching the sun climb above the garden fence and peek through the rose bushes, I know that this is a day that we'll both remember forever.

The children are up and dressing themselves quickly. Breakfast is on the table. Cereal and toast is almost more than we can manage today. There are bags still to be packed, fish to be fed, garbage to be disposed of, sheets to be changed. I'm not sure which way to run next.

"There are men with cameras across the road, Mom," Elizabeth informs me, and skips off to investigate further. Glancing through the living room sheers, I see that there are indeed a number of cameramen and reporters. They're standing, chatting together and glancing towards the house. We've never been stalked by cameras before. One could wind up feeling important.

There is a commotion in the hall below. Don's dad, mom and sister have arrived. Lonnie immediately takes Elizabeth under her wing, organizing her packing, and reducing the selection of stuffed animals to an acceptable number.

Pop and Don begin to load the bags and cases into the trunk of the car. Bob Gillingham from CBC television appears at the front door, cameraman in tow. He'd like an interview with Matthew if we wouldn't mind. Matt is only too happy to share his insights with the world.

The last suitcase is in the car, the interview over. It's seven-thirty already, and we have to leave. No time for goodbyes to Transformers in the playroom or elephants on wallpaper, to a treasured bicycle, or to soft animal friends waiting patiently in his bedroom. Or maybe, being at least as wise as we, he has said his goodbyes in his own quiet way.

Just before 8 a.m., we arrive at Hudson General, a small terminal at the south end of Vancouver International Airport. Lonnie's son Mark has already arrived. The two early-bird camera crews have followed us through the Deas Tunnel and across No. 3 Road to reach Sea Island. More cameras and reporters are in the waiting area. I recognize CKVU's Rick Hoogendoorn from our recent meeting. He asks for a brief interview if it's all right with me. It most certainly is! I'd love to utter something profound and meaningful for the evening news. However, eloquence eludes me this morning; much to my chagrin, "We're very excited" is all I can muster. Rick tries a different angle. "We're very excited," I repeat, pathetically. So much for dreams of stardom!

A sleek, shiny Lear jet stands on the runway in front of the terminal building. The three crew members stand talking by the steps.

"Did you see your plane, Matt?" Don asks, pointing to the window.

"Is that it, Dad? WOW! It's awesome."

The modest waiting room is bustling with activity. Every few minutes, the doors swing open and more friends arrive. We had no idea that they were all coming. Shirley has brought an enormous picnic basket full of cold cuts, cheeses, crackers, fruit, drinks, candies, and home-baked muffins, and even some beautiful roses. They've thought of everything.

Mr. Townsend and Mr. McCallum are here representing the Lions. We both thank them for the financial help they've offered.

Martti Huttunen rushes in dressed for a day in the world of business.

"Just wanting to make sure that everything is all right," he says.

"Come and meet the pilots," Don calls in a free moment. The three men are being kept busy. They've welcomed all the children on board. About a dozen of them are whooping and chattering, taking turns in the pilots' seats and exploring all the nooks and crannies of the compact little jet. Matt is referring to "my plane" in an unusually loud voice. This is his party. Today the spotlight is all his.

Jim, the chief pilot, is more than helpful, and co-pilots Bruce and Devery are obviously cast from the same mold. No worries here; we're in the best of hands.

An ambulance arrives shortly before 9 a.m. and comes to a stop next to the jet. Two men jump out and begin unloading medical equipment onto the plane, with help and supervision from Jim.

The children, now back in the waiting area, are beginning to show signs of restlessness. But it doesn't last for long. Margi has brought along a quartz crystal suspended from a string, which attracts them all like bees to a honey-pot.

"You mean it answers questions?" Greg asks.

"Simple questions, yes. It goes round in a circle if the answer is no, and backwards and forwards if the answer is yes.

"Ask it if it's sunny out today," Andrea suggests. Margi complies, and to the childrens' great amazement, the crystal swings gently backwards and forwards.

"Ask it if I've had my breakfast," from Austen (who obviously hasn't!). The crystal obliges, moving in a circle from Margi's motionless hand. Bug-eyed and incredulous — the children watch in silence.

"You see, it's very clever," Margi says.

Matthew is next.

"If it's so smart, get it to spell hippopotamus," he says and throws his head back, and laughs and laughs.

Shortly afterwards, Jim comes in to tell us all is ready. It's time to leave. The reporters and cameramen are out on the tarmac enjoying the morning sunshine. Matt's young friends line up along the window, their noses pressed against it as if for a better view. Elizabeth is with them. Her chin trembles, and there are tears in her eyes.

"Goodbye, sweetheart. We'll miss you. Have a wonderful summer," we tell her.

Our friends are lined up, too. Not intentionally — it just seems to happen that way. Don and I move from one to the other, hugging and kissing these special people.

"Good luck."

"Take care."

"We'll be thinking of you."

"We'll be praying for you."

Matt runs ahead and up the steps of "his" plane. He stops at the doorway and turns to smile at his friends. Cameras roll and click. Another wave, and he disappears from view. Don and I follow him across the tarmac.

"Goodbye," the men from the media call. "Good luck."

Andrew Macnab extends a hand in greeting and Jeff Vachon follows suit.

"We already know Matthew from his time in I.C.U.," says Andrew. "Hello, Matthew. Come and sit with us for take-off." The medics sit opposite each other, and Matt sits next to Andrew.

"Now, Matthew," the doctor explains, "we need to check your oxygen level, and we'll need to use some equipment. The good news is that nothing will hurt. All right?" He produces a small object that looks for all the world like a plastic clothes peg, and gently clips it onto Matt's finger.

"There," he says, "that's no problem, is it? The other thing we're going to use is very like a band-aid — it just sticks onto your skin." Jeff produces a small electrode which Matt examines minutely.

"We'll put it on your chest, Matthew," Andrew tells him. "Here, let me help you with your shirt."

Don and I sit on the other side. Through the small round window, I can see the men on the tarmac, and, just beyond, our friends and family crowding at the window. Jim speaks to the younger pilots, then turns and checks with Andrew that everyone's ready to go. He belts himself into a forward seat as the engines roar their farewell. A myriad of hands wave from the terminal as the plane taxis toward the runway.

The dark waters of the Strait of Georgia shimmer in the morning sunshine. Cars, like black ants, inch across the Lions Gate Bridge. Goodbye, Stanley Park, goodbye, Vancouver. We'll be back again. Hopefully, we'll all be back again. . .

"How's it going?" Jim asks, leaning over the seat to observe the medics at work.

"He's great. Aren't you, Matthew? We've got no problems at all. What's our elevation at present?"

"We're at about 15,000 feet. If it's OK with you, we'll head up to 20, and check back with you then. It'll sure help our fuel consumption if we can take her up higher." Then, "Just shout if you have any problems." I daydream in my corner, scarcely able to comprehend the past week's events.

Nothing seems real. I feel as if I'm floating in a bubble, and maybe the bubble will burst.

The scenery is exquisite. Snow-capped mountains, crystal-clear lakes, forests sporting all shades of green, and resplendent valleys — the small plane skims over them, treating us to breathtaking vistas.

"Sandwich, anyone?" Jim asks, rummaging through a large hamper. "Cold meats? Cheese? Danish pastry? Muffins? Fruit? Drinks? The chief pilot is not only medical coordinator, but purser and flight attendant, too. I may add that the service is unrivalled anywhere."

"Help yourself," he invites, watching Matthew eye a container of nuts. "That's what they're there for." He lowers his voice conspiratorially: "You can tell what class you're travelling by the nuts, you know." Matt's brow wrinkles as it does when something puzzles him.

"First-class gets mixed nuts. Second-class gets peanuts," Jim explains with a straight face. Matt peers meaningfully into the container — then grins broadly at his host.

Within a few hours, the view from the windows changes drastically. Magnificent mountains and forests have given way to the vast, rolling farmlands of northern B.C., and now, over the Northwest Territories, the terrain is different again. Flat but rocky, the landscape is dotted with shimmering lakes and small, stunted spruce and pine trees. The plane descends over the immense cold expanse of Great Slave Lake and prepares to land at Yellowknife. It's something of a surprise to see a moderate-sized modern town emerging from this barren northern wilderness.

"Good, Matthew," Jeff says, as the plane hits the runway. "No changes at all on the way down. You can take the clip off your finger now."

The ramp off the runway, Jim tells us, belongs to the company that owns the plane. We come to a halt close to the buildings. A refuelling truck stands by, awaiting our arrival.

"About twenty minutes," says Jim, looking at his watch. "Washrooms are by the offices. Watch your step now, won't you?"

The air is clean and cool. There's a strange feeling of space and solitude, of emptiness and nothingness. No one argues with the elements up here.

The next leg of our journey takes us over some of the world's most inhospitable terrain. Within an hour of leaving Yellowknife, we cross the Arctic Circle, and for seemingly endless thousands of miles we fly over the desolate territory of the polar regions. This is a land of barren icefields, awesome glaciers and frozen seas, home to polar bears, arctic foxes and muskoxen. Very few people live here; only the hardy Inuit with their centuries of knowledge of living with, and on, the land. The plane flies low over the unyielding rock and ice of Baffin Island, crosses Baffin Bay — and finally on to our second fuel stop, Greenland.

"Do people really live here, Mom?" Matt asks, as we fly into Sondre Stromfjord on the south west coast.

Jim opens the door and we file out into the chilly evening air. It's 8 p.m. local time — we've been travelling for almost seven hours — but thanks to the midnight sun, it is broad daylight. We scurry along the grey runway, lined on one side by the grey, rocky plateau wall. Clouds hang low, and they too are grey. Grey and cold. Greenland, for me, will forever conjure up the colour grey.

The airport building is warm and busy. There are far more men than women. They sit in groups, drinking beer or liquor and speaking a language we don't understand.

We treat Andrew and Jeff to supper — though treat is hardly the word. The food looks dull and uninspired. Some of the items are unrecognizable.

"Looks like penguin stew to me," Don jokes. "Or how about some walrus casserole?" Our Canadian money confuses the blond, blue-eyed cashier. Their Danish money confuses us. She laboriously works out the rate of exchange. She admits she doesn't know for sure, and we have no idea at all. We certainly don't come out the winners.

After supper, Don, Matt and I attempt a short walk, but neither Matt nor I can stand it for more than a minute.

It's almost time to board the plane. I've been to the restroom and am waiting for the boys to arrive. Two men and a woman are standing close by, talking and looking in my direction. One of the men comes over and speaks to me in his own language.

"Sorry. English," I say, shaking my head and smiling amiably. The man tries again. His English is thick with the accents of Denmark. I can just make out his request.

"Excuse me. You come with me. We talk. We drink. We dance. We. . ."

"Sorry," I interrupt. "Plane. We're catching a plane," and I point in the direction of the waiting jet. "Sorry."

Don is highly amused. "Boy, they must be hard up here," he chortles — perhaps a little too quickly!

On board again, Andrew and Jeff continue their careful monitoring. Matt is faring amazingly well, and the jet can climb to 30,000 feet. The pilots spell each other off, and Bruce is purser-at-large for now. We pass the time easily, reading, talking, and playing Uno with Matt. Far below us, the outside world glides by — a white, bleak, forbidding domain. Bruce comes back to talk with Andrew.

"Our plans have changed a bit," he says. "It seems that Reykjavik's fog-bound. Jim's wondering, if it's OK with you, if we could just head straight for Prestwick?" This, I think, is where we could have come unglued! Had Matt been ill; had we needed hospital care. . . But fate is on our side today. We know there will be no problem.

It is scarcely 6 a.m. when the plane puts down in Prestwick. The dawn is fresh and new — and we have it nearly all to ourselves. We find the restrooms as the plane is refuelled for the last time, and then, just before boarding, arrange a mini photo session: Matt with Jim. . . Matt with Andrew and Jeff. . . Matt with Jim, Devery and Bruce. . . Matt on his own. . .

Leaving Prestwick by six-thirty, we saunter down the length of the British Isles. A cluster of lakes sparkles like gems in the morning sun. Rugged mountains and rolling hills proudly display their grandeur. Moors and dales too quickly give way to row upon row of miniature houses with postage-stamp gardens; brown and grey, unpainted and dusty — Coronation Street and Railway Close. Over Cheshire's green plain with its dairy cattle, over pocket-sized villages with thatched cottages and neat, colourful gardens, over motorways and cities, over castles and parkland . . . For me, this is home.

"Ten minutes to Gatwick," Jim calls from the front, as Matt takes up his position next to Jeff for the final monitoring.

Magazines and Uno cards, colouring books and crayons — all accessories of the last fourteen hours — are tucked away in bags as the plane prepares to land.

Our passports are checked as we stand in the sun. Then it's time to say goodbye. Matt hugs each of the pilots in turn, while Don and I shake their hands.

"Thank you," we say. "We'll never forget what you've done for us."

The journey could not have been better: Matthew has stayed so well. Incredibly well. And now we're in England. We're where we need to be. The first hurdle is over.

Two young men stand chatting, leaning against the perimeter fence. One carries a camera slung over his shoulder. As soon as we reach the gate, they come forward and greet us.

"I'm John Wellington," the fair-haired man tells us. "Keith Morgan let us know you were coming. We're with *The Mail on Sunday*. Could we have a few pictures, and maybe a brief story?"

Jim has ordered a taxi by radio. It's there already, polished and waiting. An officious chauffeur peers at his watch, and coughs loudly every few minutes.

The interview is over. It's time for more goodbyes.

''We'll be staying in London for the weekend,'' says Andrew, ''then we'll be flying back on Monday.''

More thank-you's, more hugs, more handshakes.

''Thank you for everything,'' Matthew says. The medics turn quickly away.

Chapter Ten

The taxi is gleaming, the driver immaculate in a smart dark suit. Every hair is in place. He ceremoniously holds the doors open for us and we tumble onto plush seats with generous armrests. Don sits in the front with Charles Chauffeur. Matt and I sink into the back seat, and Matt immediately falls asleep.

"I've never seen such a well-kept taxi," Don offers by way of conversation.

"Well, we do 'ave a standard to keep up, yer know," the man replies, reaching under the dashboard for a pair of driving gloves. "Now tike me. I cleans me car for an hour each day. The kinds of people we drives expects it. We're not like ordinary taxi drivers, yer know. We're more 'ticular. We 'ave to be a cut above that to drive a private car. Now wheres exactly are yer going?"

"Connaught Road," I tell him. "It's just off Putney Hill. My sister lives . . ."

"Now tike an ordinary cabbie. 'E'd likely not know wheres that was. 'E'd likely drive 'alfways round England to get yers there. And no air conditioning on an 'ot day. And 'is cab not clean . . ." I'm engulfed by a wave of exhaustion, and, mercifully, drift off to sleep. Don is left on his own, with an unparalleled opportunity to learn about the hierarchy of Britain's cabbies.

I come to with a start. The cab has stopped. Matthew's still fast asleep, facing into the seat with his arms raised. His face is pale and his breathing irregular.

"Hon, do you remember how to get to Joan's?" Don is asking. The driver's head is buried in a road map of London.

"I'll find it in a minute. There's no problem," he's saying. His neck and ears are crimson. His embarrassment is painful.

"We need Putney Hill," I tell him. "I can find it from there. Where are we now?"

"We think we're in Fulham," Don answers, "but we're not too sure."

Matthew stirs by my side. He tries to change position but cannot breathe properly, so resumes his one safe pose. There are dark circles beneath his eyes. His nails are tinged with blue.

"Ask!" I snap. "Our son is ill."

"I'll find it in a jiffy," the miserable man replies, holding the map two inches from his nose. "If only I 'ad me other glasses. We're not far, yer know."

"Ask," I growl, my patience dissolving completely.

The traffic is backing up to our right, as it waits for the lights to change. Two London cabs draw up by our side. Our mortified driver lowers his window and calls to the closest cabbie.

"Putney 'ill. Which way?" He visibly squirms in his seat. The young cabbie grins with undisguised amusement. "Wrong way, mate," he yells. "Turn around, right at the traffic lights. You can't miss it." Our driver nods tersely. He removes his gloves and shrinks into his seat. Much to our relief, within minutes I recognize our whereabouts, and can direct the unhappy man up Putney Hill and right onto Connaught Road.

We tumble out, yanking cases, coats, and the precious picnic basket with us. Don extracts an envelope of English money from his wallet.

"Sorry, Guv. No change," I hear our chauffeur telling him, obviously not averse to using the oldest ploy in the book. Don's wallet is forty-five pounds lighter as the taxi returns to its hunting grounds, and we, the tourists, are more than a little wiser.

Joan has her own apartment on the third floor of Connaught House. In response to our ring, she quickly appears in the lobby to take stock of the situation. "Come on up," she welcomes us. "So good to see you. Let's get your things in the elevator." Matthew, despite his exhaustion, is looking better again. At least he can control his breathing when he's awake.

There's a short, narrow passageway leading into Joan's living area. It's home to her bicycle, and it doesn't occur to any of us to move it. With great care and considerable struggle, we inch our cumbersome baggage past it, moulding ourselves in and out of its contours, frequently being gouged by a pedal or handlebar.

Matthew, to my relief, falls asleep on the sofa. Joan makes coffee and toast and regales us with news and anecdotes as she works. Don and I sit slumped in our seats, laughing hysterically at images conjured up by her dry British humour. Tears trickle down our cheeks and we wallow in the pleasure of relaxing. We used to laugh a lot, but it's been a luxury now for a long time.

By 11 a.m., the day is already hot and oppressive, and neither Don nor I can keep our eyes open. Joan leaves us sleeping and heads down to the High Street to get some groceries. She returns two hours later, laden with cold cuts and salads from Marks and Spencers and Sainsbury's.

"It's stifling out there today," she says, putting down the bags and resting on the back of a chair. "I can't imagine how anyone will play tennis in this. Oh, did you know that Wimbledon is on this week?" We didn't know, but are pleased.

"Great. That'll help to pass some time. Matt loves to play tennis. Maybe he'll enjoy watching it too."

We all observe the little boy who loves to play tennis. He must have stirred at some point, and removed his shirt, which now lies by his feet. He is half-sitting, half-lying on the sofa. His body is twisted so his head can rest on his arms, which are supported by the raised arm of the sofa. From the strange movements of his back and chest, it is easy to see that his breathing is grossly abnormal. Don and I are as used to this as we will ever be, but Joan has had no practice.

"Are you sure he's all right?" she asks, obviously alarmed.

"He's OK," Don reassures her. "Sleeping is always a problem." It's at moments like this that I know we're not acting a minute too soon.

We leave Matt to rest while we eat some lunch. There's so much to talk about. So much to tell from Canada — almost totally connected with Matt's illness — and so much to catch up on with my own family here. Things are not good. Illness and marriage problems are plaguing my brother's and sisters' families. It's apparently been a black year for us all.

We have to leave. We need to get settled, and above all, to sleep. Joan has phoned Mrs. King, who's expecting us this afternoon. Joan phones for a taxicab, (one of the average, second-class variety) and we gather up our son, bags, cases and picnic basket, and inch our way once more around the offending Raleigh.

The cabbie is as black as night. Sweat glistens on his brow. He watches silently as we heave and haul our baggage into the cab.

"Phone me when you're settled," Joan calls. "I'll let Mum know you've arrived."

"Harefield Hospital, please," Don tells the driver as he climbs in beside him. Matthew is asleep in seconds. The same position. The same laboured breathing. The same chilling pallor. I watch him for a few minutes, and marvel again at his courage. He never complains. Never whines or clings. It's as though he accepts that this is his lot — and he'll just do the best he can.

Ah, London. What a magnificent city! Buckingham Palace, St. Paul's, Big Ben, Harrod's, Hyde Park — the list is endless. Steeped in history and tradition, it's truly a tourist's delight. It is not, however, this side of London which we are treated to on this hot Saturday afternoon. We careen from one grimy, litter-strewn High Street into another, encircling London's East End.

Plump women clad in gaudy sundresses browse through the wares of street-markets. Scruffy dogs roam free, cringing around the stalls and fouling the sidewalks. Horns sound constantly, as cars manoeuvre through crowds of heedless shoppers, vying for space in the narrow streets. This is a far cry indeed from the usual beats of London visitors.

In less than an hour, we're in the country. The cabbie takes this as a cue to drive even faster, and we swing past fields and hedgerows at an alarming rate, narrowly missing oncoming traffic. The scenery changes again. Houses rise from the fields to our left; an ancient church can be glimpsed to our right.

"Which part of Harefield?" The driver's clipped Caribbean accent breaks through the silence. Don awakens abruptly.

"The hospital," he replies. "We're staying at Sanctuary Close, which is apparently near the hospital gates." We're in another High Street now, but this is much cleaner and less crowded than the ones we've just been through. We swing around the roundabout, with its old pub on one side and the village green on the other. The road forks and we bear left, and suddenly we're here. A large wooden sign declares that this is, indeed, Harefield Hospital. Looking up the driveway, we can make out a moderate-sized, two-storey brick building. There's nothing to mark it as special in any way. Thank goodness Susan Shallcross had told us:

"It's in a village. In spite of the work they do there, it doesn't look special at all. And they tend to be short of basic things — I'd take your own towels, for example." She's right about it not looking special! We decide to reserve judgement. This place, after all, is Matthew's only hope. We have nowhere else to go.

The driver follows the road to the right, and within minutes we're parked in Sanctuary Close. The cabbie's sharp eyes pick out the door we need.

"Wake up, Matthew, we're here," I tell him, shaking him gently. His eyes open. He scoops up Doggy and is quickly out of the taxi. Don pays the driver, who roars from the close at the same unnerving speed.

Ruth King is a slight lady, somewhere in her sixties.

"You must be tired. Let me take that bag," she insists, leading us up the three flights of stairs.

"You have the whole of the top floor to yourself. There's a bedroom here, and one at the end of the corridor. This is the bathroom, and there's a kettle and tea and coffee in the cupboard if you want a drink at night. Breakfast is generally around eight. You can get food in the hospital canteen, mind you, but I wouldn't recommend it." Mrs. King pulls a face that speaks volumes.

"That good, eh?" jokes Don. She nods and grimaces.

"If you need anything, just ask, won't you?"

We're exhausted, and the heat is stifling. But we're here. The relief is overwhelming. Sanctuary Close is well named.

The next morning, we're all wide awake by 6 a.m., victims of the inevitable jet-lag. The room is still warm from yesterday's heat, and the rays of morning sunshine warn of another sweltering day. Don lies in bed, munching on a muffin and reading a thriller. Matt is lounging on the floor, giving his Transformers an early morning workout. The room is comfortable and homey. Flower-patterned wallpaper collides with a contrasting carpet. Both join forces to clash with the gaily adorned bedspreads. The final result is surprising. The room is like a good friend — welcoming, cheerful and relaxing. Matthew's room, at the end of the corridor, is almost its twin, and the bathroom, while less colourful, offers the same affable hospitality. The cooing of doves is all that breaks the silence of the sleepy village morning. There is time to dream, to reflect, to take stock.

A long, contented time passes before we hear the first sounds of movement from downstairs. The cough is rasping and gravelly, racking its owner for several minutes. And then the tantalizing smell of fresh-brewed coffee wafts up the stairway. Matthew, fully dressed, departs for the kitchen to inspect Mrs. King for himself. Don and I dress quickly, and follow our son downstairs.

"Come on in. Come and sit," she invites, as we appear at her kitchen door. Then, "Lie down, 'Dhesia. Bad girl," to the tan Rhodesian ridgeback who has risen to check us out. Mrs. King has dark rings beneath her eyes. A cigarette burns in the ashtray on the kitchen counter.

"Don't mind me in the morning," she admonished us. "I feel like a scarecrow till I've had my coffee and cigarette." She coughs again — the low, bronchial cough of a chronic smoker.

"Now what are you going to have? I cook breakfast on Sunday. On other days, there's cereal, toast and fruit. Is that all right?" We assure her that will be just fine.

"I'm not a morning person either, Mrs. King," I tell her. "So long as I get a big mug of coffee, anything is fine with me."

Mrs. King is a mine of information. She has worked with the Hospital for a number of years, offering bed and breakfast to families like ourselves.

"There's free accommodation in the hospital grounds," she tells us, "but Matthew has to be an inpatient before you're eligible for that. When do you see the big man himself?" she enquires, referring, of course, to the eminent Mr. Murad.

"We're expected tomorrow morning," Don answers, "but it's for

Matthew to be assessed. I wouldn't think we'll see him then." Mrs. King agrees.

"He's a very busy man. He operates at several different hospitals, and the transplants are often at night. I've heard that the best time to catch him is in the wee hours of the morning, between operations." For some strange reason, we find this snippet amusing. It all goes with the territory somehow!

The walk down to the village is probably no more than a quarter of a mile, but Matthew finds it difficult today.

The village itself is large and relatively unkempt. We can hardly believe the state of the green. Papers of every size and colour are strewn across the grass. There are two large wastebaskets, proof that some effort has been made, but they're both stuffed to the brim, and can only stand uselessly by as the overflow mounts.

I leave Don to push his son on the swings, and hurry away in search of a Sunday newspaper. All the shops are closed today, with the exception, of course, of the news agents. Sunday papers, after all, are a tradition in England. Every taste is catered to, from the vicious gossip of the gutter press to the lofty editorials of the *Times* and *Guardian*. The papers are piled on the counter with the "low-lifes" at one end and the "intellectuals" at the other. Somewhere in the middle is *The Mail on Sunday*. The photo is extremely good. Matt is sitting on the sidewalk, smiling and waving. "Flight of hope for lung-boy Matthew," the caption reads, and underneath is a short version of the story of his illness and the trip from Canada.

"Well, you're a star, guy," I call to Matt, having rushed back to the village green. Don reads the article aloud while Matt looks at the photo. He grunts nonchalantly before moving onto the next item of business.

"Hey, Mom, let's go and phone Granny Petal." There's a kiosk at the corner of the green. The glass is broken, but the phone still works. Mum is waiting for our call. She cannot hide the strain from her voice. We reassure her as best we can: "At least we're here, Mum, and Matt is doing well."

It's Matthew's turn now.

"Hello, Granny Petal . . ." They talk for several minutes and when he hands the receiver back to me, he's all smiles.

"Granny's got twenty dollars for me — and some bubble gum!"

It's already one-thirty, and we're ravenous. We soon discover, however, that apart from the pubs, there's little choice in places to eat. We go for The Tandoori, a small Indian restaurant close to the village green. Matt picks at his rice and chapatis in his usual uninterested manner. We've long since given up nagging. We know he isn't hungry.

The day is as hot as anticipated. Back at Mrs. King's we all fall asleep on our beds.

We're awakened by a noise on the stairs — footsteps and talking — and then a knock on the door.

"Are you awake? There's a visitor for you!" Mrs. King calls. The door opens and my sister Brenda appears. We hug each other, both laughing and talking at once.

"What are you doing here? Did you drive down?" It turns out that she has indeed driven all the way down from Cheshire in their best car. They would like us to have it while we're staying here. They think we'll need it, being out in a village.

"Thanks so much, Bren. It'll be marvellous to have wheels."

Unfortunately, Bren has to leave immediately to catch her train back to Cheshire, so we pile into the car and race for Watford Junction. The drive back from Watford is unnerving, to say the least. Don seems compelled to navigate each and every roundabout in the wrong direction. We are a danger to pedestrians and a menace to the British motorist. It's obvious that we'll need a lot of practice at driving on the "wrong" side.

Matthew settles to sleep early, but Don and I lie awake for a long time. The old fears have returned; the nagging doubts, the "what ifs." Finally, hot and exhausted, we fall into a fitful sleep . . .

. . . the noise is deafening. Something is coming through the roof. My heart is pounding. I'm wide awake now and ready to flee.

"You awake, hon?" Don hisses. In the darkness, I can just make out his form by the window.

"What on earth was that?" I demand, somewhat braver now that the noise has abated.

"A helicopter." Don cannot disguise his excitement.

"They must be doing a transplant. Remember what Mrs. King said? The organs often come in at night." The numbers glow on the clock by Don's bed. Half past two . . . and someone is about to get a second chance at life.

We awake to the smell of Mrs. King's coffee, and the sounds of chatting in the kitchen below.

"Hear the chopper?" Mrs. King asks excitedly as we enter. "Matthew was just asking all about it, weren't you, Matthew? I was telling him that the doctors sometimes use it to pick up patients." She turns her back to Matt and pointedly catches Don's eye. Her expression asks the questions. Don nods reassuringly. We don't want to deceive our son, but neither do we want him burdened. Another child must die before Matt can have his surgery. At six years old, he shouldn't have to cope with that. "Where do the helicopters land, Mrs. King?'' Don asks, reaching for another piece of toast.

"At the side of the hospital," she answers, "there's a flat, grassy area where they come down. There are no lights yet, though," she adds, "so when they're expecting one in at night, they light the area up with the headlights from three cars. What are you going to eat, Matthew? Come on now . . . have a banana.''

We are incredulous. Patients flock from every corner of the globe because of Harefield's reputation. Its chief surgeon is renowned for his brilliant pioneering surgery. Dedication and excellence are the cornerstones. Miracles are wrought here . . . and car headlights are used to guide in the helicopters!

Breakfast is over. It's time to leave for the hospital. The morning is foggy, but promises to be another hot day. We walk through the parking area and down a narrow passageway. Along a sidewalk, we catch the scent of roses and honeysuckle from hidden gardens. Across the road and we're at the metal gates of Harefield Hospital.

The lobby is small and unassuming. That's probably not the right word: renovations are in progress, and the whole place is a mess. Two workmen sit on a pile of boards at the edge of the rubble, surrounded by dust and debris and the tools of their trade. An extremely pleasant lady, obviously displaced from her usual quarters, sits behind a makeshift desk to the right-hand side. As we approach, she smiles warmly. "The children's ward? That's P.S.U. Just follow that corridor and then keep right. You'll pass the new construction and the operating rooms. At the end of the corridor, turn left, and you're into P.S.U. All right?''

It's only 8 a.m. but the Paediatric Surgical Unit is already bustling with people. It's located in an old part of the hospital, and is basically a long corridor with rooms off to each side. The nurses' office isn't difficult to recognize. A tall, dark-haired nurse greets us at the door. It's obvious that Sister Hill is busy, and she quickly directs us to the end of the corridor.

"Please, would you wait in the parents' lounge," she asks. "Someone will see to you as soon as we have a minute.'' The lounge is adequate. For some reason, it is two connecting rooms, one small and one medium-sized. All the usual trappings of a waiting area are there — sofa, chairs, coffee table, and, of course, the inevitable television. The smaller room is sparsely furnished — a few chairs, a small fridge for parents' food, and a couple of folding beds. There is also an unexpected convenience: a telephone is mounted on the wall. A woman speaks into it in high, excited tones, in a language neither of us can understand. She waves her free arm expressively through the air, then grasps dramatically at her forehead. Her voice becomes quiet, almost a moan. Perched on another of the chairs is an East Indian woman in a brightly coloured sari. She nods and smiles briefly before resuming her anxious surveillance in the direction of the children's rooms. A young man sits on the sofa rocking a fragile-looking girl on his lap. The child is blond, with pale-blue eyes and pallid skin. Her lips are blue, as are the ends of her club-shaped fingers. A tall, curly-haired woman sits close to them reading a children's story aloud. She stops abruptly in mid-sentence.

"Are you for assessment, too?" she asks.

"Yes," replies Don. "We're hoping that our son can have a heart/lung transplant. Is that why you're here?"

"It's all that's left for Emma now," she says, taking the child's hand in her own. "They've tried everything else." We are immediately close to Sue and Nigel Braley. We exchange our children's medical histories, worry about the assessment, and discuss "the wait." Matt appears at the door with a toy in hand. He's found the playroom and is feeling quite at home.

"He doesn't look ill enough," Nigel says, almost to himself.

"You'd never know he was sick," Sue adds, "just look at him." We all turn to study the little boy. His blue eyes sparkle, and his cheeks are round and rosy. He's laughing heartily. Few could detect the flaw in his breathing. I'm gripped with doubt again. Maybe this remission will last for weeks, or even months. Or who knows, even years. Maybe we should wait . . .

It's ten o'clock before a young staff nurse arrives at the door and calls Matthew's name purposefully. She leads us to one of the children's rooms and takes some routine information. Matt is temporarily assigned one of the two beds. In the other a beautiful dark-skinned child cries softly. The East Indian lady with whom we had shared the lounge is sitting on the bed, comforting him.

"You going to be all right, little one. You going to be well now."

The door opens and Sister Hill enters with a tall, powerfully built man wearing a dark-blue suit. They stand with their backs toward us, facing the weeping child. The mother looks up at the sound of Sister Hill's voice. She sees the man, then, much to our amazement, leaps from the bed to face the visitor. A torrent of broken English pours out from her lips.

"Thank you. Thank you. You save my boy. He going to die, and now he live. His heart no good. Now it well. How can I thank you?" Her eyes are brimming with tears of emotion. The child stops weeping, distracted by the scene before him. He stares in amazement as his excited mother babbles on, all but threatening to embrace the big man.

"We're very happy with his progress," I hear him say, as he backs toward the door.

"Thank you. Thank you. I cannot thank you enough, Mr. Murad . . ."

Mr. Murad. *The* Mr. Murad? The one we have travelled five thousand miles to see? Now it's my turn to get excited! Don't we even get to say "Hello"? A pleasant young doctor appears at the bedside. He introduces himself as Dr. Jensen, and explains that he is the registrar for Dr. Richmond, the paediatric cardiology consultant. He tells us they will order the tests that Matthew must undergo before being accepted as a transplant candidate.

"The tests generally take a week to complete," he tells us. "Today, he'll have X-rays taken, as well as an ECG and an echocardiogram. All right?" he asks, smiling hesitantly.

The young nurse appears at the bedside. "Did anyone show you round yet?" Then, in response to our shaking heads, "No! Come on, then. I'll show you where everything is. There's not much — it's only a small unit — but it helps to know your way about. I'm Abbie, by the way. We'll start at this end." We turn right out of the doorway, and follow Abbie up the corridor. She pauses at the door of a four-bed room. "This is I.C.U.," she says. The sounds are all familiar: monitors softly beeping, suction tubes gurgling, the purr of respirators, and the unnatural silence of young children. We pass the nurses' office and Abbie stops again.

"And this is the transplant room," she tells us, opening the door to a rather ordinary-looking room. "They come back here after surgery. As you can see, it's empty at present." Don and I are transfixed. This is where much of Matt's battle will be fought.

"Beep, beep!"

"Be careful, Charlotte, mind where you're going now." Another accent, but at least it's understandable! Its owner, an attractive blond woman, holds onto the offending tricycle, apologizing profusely.

"No problem," we tell her. "No one got hurt." And they move on, the thin, pale child pedalling with grim determination.

"That's Charlotte Grant," Abbie volunteers, leading us toward the patio. "She had a heart/lung transplant about three weeks ago. She's had some ups and downs, but she's doing fine now." She points toward a path skirting the huge lawn. "If you want to go into the village . . ." But I hear nothing more. That little girl. She's had a transplant too. It can work. Life can be normal again. We know the statistics, but some things have to be seen to be believed. A new heart and lungs just three weeks ago — and she's riding a trike. The warm glow of hope surges through me; Don catches my eye and winks.

"Hey, Matthew." He stoops to talk with his son. "That little girl on the trike had the same operation that you're going to have. And it was only three weeks ago. What do you think of that?"

Matt responds with the "in" word for six- year-olds, "Awesome."

The day passes easily enough. The tests are all familiar and painless. By

2 p.m. we're free to leave, to wander down to the village to open a bank account and stock up on groceries. We spend the rest of the day exploring the surrounding towns.

The following morning we're once more at P.S.U. by eight. The unit is hectic, and we're again assigned to the parents' lounge. Charlotte Grant and her parents occupy the main sofa, Charlotte sitting between them, listening intently while her mother reads a story. We introduce ourselves, and within minutes the children amble next door to the playroom. Barry and Clare Grant, it turns out, are from New Zealand. They're a young, intelligent, articulate couple who radiate an amazing optimism and strength. The story they have to tell is any parent's nightmare: cruel, tragic and totally unfair.

Charlotte, Clare tells us, was born in October 1980, making her now three months shy of six. When she was only a week old, her brother, Oliver, then twenty-one months old, collapsed and was subsequently admitted to Greenlane Hospital, Auckland's main cardiac centre. To the specialist's experienced eyes and touch, Oliver's condition appeared ominous.

"I think we have big trouble here," he said. "A cardiac catheterization will have to be done to confirm my diagnosis." That was the beginning of the Grants' life with pulmonary hypertension. Oliver's pulmonary veins were hardening over the lungs, restricting the blood flow and overworking his heart. He was already in cardiac failure, and it was too late to do anything other than try to keep him comfortable. Clare and Barry watched him grow weaker day by day, until finally, eleven months after the initial diagnosis, Oliver died. He was two years and eight months old.

One month later, the Grants celebrated Charlotte's first birthday. The small blond child took her first steps to mark the occasion. But then, incredibly, the familiar symptoms appeared: hesitation on climbing stairs; breathlessness; sweatiness and clamminess on slight exertion. Barry and Clare couldn't believe it. An insidious fear wove through their raw grief for Oliver. Instinctively, they knew that Charlotte would be a victim too.

"You won't believe this, though." Clare sits on the front edge of her seat. Her face is flushed. "The doctors say it's not hereditary. The odds of it happening to a family twice are too long to contemplate." The inevitable "Why us?" had turned, understandably, to "Why us again?" It was back to "one day at a time" for the Grants, back to uncertainty and fear, and the inevitable grasping at hope. Charlotte fared better than her brother. She was stronger, a fighter, never ceasing to amaze those who cared for her. Her good fortune, however, had run out in February of this year. She had contracted a lethal virus and became extremely ill. The memory of it is almost too painful for Barry.

"We doubted she'd ever get out of hospital," he says, still horrified by the experience.

"Anyway," Clare breaks in, "it was then that I happened to buy an Australian Women's Weekly from the hospital coffee shop. And there it was, on the front page — the story of an Australian girl with pulmonary hypertension who had gone to England for a heart/lung transplant. I was so excited." Clare had raced down the corridor to find Charlotte's doctor.

"It's too new . . . experimental . . . only done a few." Clare wasn't deterred. They had already lost one child. They had nothing to lose and everything to gain. She phoned the Australian girl's mother and asked dozens of questions. The doctor, impressed by their determination, applied for special funding, and made arrangements with Harefield. On April 10, they flew out of Auckland in search of a new life for Charlotte.

Once in England, they had settled down to wait for donor organs to become available. It was eight weeks later, at the Harefield Hospital fete, that the beeper in Clare's bag went off. Clare's heart sunk with apprehension, but the frail little girl at her side laughed, sang and danced with glee. At last she was going to have the chance to be like her friends back home in New Zealand, to run and climb, to swim and dance.

The operation took five hours. Twenty-four hours later she was off the respirator, breathing by herself with the new lungs.

"I'll never forget the sight," Clare continues. "Long, slow breathing. Very shaky. And the scarlet colour gone from her lips, ears and fingers. It was incredible." Four days after the operation, Charlotte was up and walking. They know they must take it a day at a time — but, so far, things are going well.

"Can Matthew come now?" Sister Hill asks from the doorway. "They want to fit him with a twenty-four-hour heart monitor."

"It doesn't hurt, Matthew," Charlotte pipes up. "I had that. It's only tape on your chest." And sure enough, it's just as Charlotte has promised.

Our second day at Harefield is over. We're ravenous, and it's time for supper. We drive to a small town some five miles away, and find an Italian restaurant with a promising menu. Matt is asleep in the car, in his usual position — sitting up and facing against the back seat. He looks peaceful, temporarily removed from illness, tests and uncertainty.

The restaurant is empty except for two waiters busily setting tables for the evening. One steps forward to greet us.

"Our son is ill and sleeping in the car. Would it be possible to eat outside?" Don asks.

"For you, signor, anything is possible," the man replies. He clears a table of its cutlery, hauls it through the door, and deposits it on the sidewalk.

He disappears into the gloom of the restaurant, quickly returning with a white linen cloth, which he spreads on the table with a flourish. The cutlery is reset, candles are lit with ceremony, and finally, a small vase of flowers completes his artistry.

"Signora." The waiter bows deeply and with a showy gesture ushers me into a chair.

"Signor." He repeats the performance for Don, before rushing to offer the menu. Other patrons stare in surprise. We hear the waiter turn down their requests.

"Sorry. Their child is ill. They have to watch him."

The evening air is warm and soft. I can see the small brown head resting against the seat. It's still and peaceful. We sip our wine, enjoying each moment while we may. Seafood fettucini never tasted so good.

Wednesday, July 2

Matthew's not so well today. It's nothing you can put your finger on, but he's tired and quiet. The friendly receptionist greets us cheerfully as we pass through the front lobby. Then along the corridor and past the construction site for the new I.C.U. There is evidence of progress — a large pile of bricks has been moved from one corner to another. Faces on P.S.U. are becoming familiar now; some even have names attached to them. In the end cubicle, a tall, handsome man keeps vigil over a tiny baby. He speaks no English, just nods and smiles. His eyes are sad and troubled, rarely leaving the motionless bundle lying in the crib.

Matthew is to have blood work done today, and also some pulmonary function tests. These are nothing new for him, and he still has plenty of free time to play and make new friends. We wander out to the patio and relax in the morning sunshine.

"Hello, are you the Ekroths?" The dark-haired woman calling from the doorway is probably close to our age. She clutches a folder and a pen, and looks decidedly official.

"I'm Diane Kent," she starts, extending a hand in greeting. "I'm the transplant coordinator for Mr. Murad's team. I know young Matthew hasn't finished his assessment yet, but I need to complete his forms. Beautiful weather, isn't it?"

Don rises to offer his seat, and pulls up another chair for himself. We're soon deep in conversation. We have so many questions, so much to learn. Diane, it seems, has nearly all the answers. She starts by telling us something about herself. She's a registered nurse and midwife and has been at Harefield for thirteen years. Her job initially was to set up the homograft department, for the preparation of human aortic valves for implantation. She saw it as an interesting change from regular nursing. It was in that same year that Mr. Murad performed his first heart transplant at Harefield. (Christian Barnard had, of course, pioneered the surgery in 1967 in South Africa, but shortly afterward, a voluntary moratorium was imposed on further operations until more was known about the treatment and prevention of rejection. Six years later, the program was ready to run again.)

Diane had frequently needed to send valves around the world, and was well versed in world airlines, customs and immigration, and carrier services, so she was given the task of hiring helicopters and small planes at a moment's notice for the retrieval of donor organs. The coordinator side of her job was a self-developed enterprise. There was no formal training. She had to develop the routines by trial and error, and by building good relationships with donor hospitals and the transplant services here and throughout Europe.

We learn that Matt's donor organs may come from the U.K. or from one of many countries in Europe. The U.K. Transplant Service in Bristol was originally the computer-matching centre for all kidney donors and patients. For the last five years, all transplant patients have also been registered on this computer. When a donor becomes available anywhere in the U.K., the relevant information is fed to the computer, which, in turn, finds the most suitable recipients for heart, lungs, liver and kidneys. The service then contacts the units concerned. There are similar services in Scandinavia, France, Italy and Spain. Eurotransplant covers Belgium, Holland and West Germany, and the British patients are registered with all of these services. However, Diane goes on to explain, in practice, many hospitals with donor organs to offer contact Harefield directly, because of its size and reputation.

"Well, surely there can't be much of a wait, then," Don interjects. "Between the millions of people who live in the U.K. and the cooperation of all the European countries, there must be plenty of organs!"

"There should be plenty of organs, but there aren't," Diane answers simply. "Generally speaking, healthy people don't want to think about dying, so they don't take the necessary few minutes to fill out a donor card and make their wishes known to their next of kin. If death comes suddenly, as is often the case with, say, a young person killed in a car accident, the family are often too distraught and shocked to think about organ donation. And the medical staff, unless specially trained, don't like to approach them on such a sensitive subject. I'm afraid there are never enough organs, and sometimes people die while waiting. It can be terribly hard."

Diane pulls a form from the folder and starts to write. "Where will you be staying once the assessment is completed?" she asks. I give her Mum's name and address in Cheshire.

"How would you travel back to the hospital once there are organs?"

"Probably by car," Don tells her.

"How long will it take?"

"About four hours, I'd guess, allowing for a hitch or two."

"Four hours . . ." she mutters, never lifting her head. She finishes writing and checks the form again.

"Good, I think that's it for the moment. We'll be giving you a pager, or a 'bleep' as we call them, which must be kept turned on at all times. The call could come anytime, night or day. Also, you should keep a bag packed, so that you're ready to leave immediately." Diane glances at her watch, and gathers up her folder. "Have I missed anything? Did you have any other questions?"

"What are his chances? Will he get on the list?" Don asks for us both.

"Don't worry about it," she smiles. "I can't know for sure, but I can tell you that if there's any chance of success, Mr. Murad will do his best to give young Matthew that chance. I must fly. I've another family to see. I'll be around again tomorrow. Bye for now." And she disappears through the corridor doors.

Thursday, July 3

Matt is scheduled only for chest measurements today. I'm not sure why the assessment takes five days when two would surely be enough, but there's probably an explanation, and I'm not about to make waves. The chest measurement is quite simply that. There is some leeway with the size of the donor heart, but not so with the lungs. They have to fit inside the rib cage. There can be no mistakes.

By 10 a.m. we're free for the day. Matthew's present from Granny Petal arrives in the morning mail. He'd love to go shopping to check out England's Transformers! We borrow a wheelchair from Northwood Red Cross, and drive to a nearby shopping centre. Fenwick's offers an appetizing lunch menu. Matt picks at his food, of course. "Never mind," I think, "we'll be up at Mum's by tomorrow evening." I can well imagine her stocking up on food supplies — a slightly stooped, determined figure, filling up endless baskets at Marks and Spencers. And the candy tin will be overflowing, with surplus bars and bags piled on top of the fridge. I can hardly wait to get home. To see family and friends once more. To relax and share our burden. To be someone's child again, and be taken care of. It will be such a special time!

The toy shop in Boots has the exact transformers that Matt's looking for. He climbs out of the wheelchair long enough to select and pay for them. People, especially children, stare at the wheelchair with its young occupant. Matt doesn't seem to mind, although he carefully avoids eye contact. But there's a resignation, a kind of acceptance that this is his lot. And, after all, it's not all bad!

It's evening when we arrive back at Mrs. King's. Her face lights up at seeing Matthew.

"Had a good time, did you?" she asks, and is treated to a display of the Transformers.

"They make up the rest of Bruticus," Matt explains. "Now I've got all the parts." Mrs. King grins and nods, as though it all makes sense.

"There was a phone call for you," she says, reaching for the telephone pad. She reads verbatim from her notes, her face flushed with excitement.

"A Mr. Roy McMurtry, an official of the Canadian government (in fact, the Canadian High Commissioner), phoned at two-forty p.m. from B.C. House. On behalf of the Canadian government, he wants to know if he can assist you in any way." Mrs. King finishes reading and positively beams at us all. Even Matt understands the honour.

"Wow," he says, his eyes dancing.

"Wow" indeed! Even the Canadian government is rooting for this little boy! A warmth engulfs us. Our strength is renewed. Surely we cannot fail.

It's nine o'clock and I'm running the water for Matt's bath. He's tired but happy. The two new Transformers, and anticipation at seeing Granny Petal again, have greatly boosted his spirits.

"Lean forward, guy, and I'll wash your hair," I tell him. He seems a little more breathless than usual. He's probably just tired, I think. He's clean and warm and cuddly as we tuck him into bed, propping him up against the large mound of pillows.

But he doesn't settle. No position is comfortable. We try different tactics: light on, light off; window open, window closed; sitting with him, going back to bed. Nothing makes a difference. Somehow, we manage to stay calm. We've had so much practice at quelling panic, it's almost second nature. Almost. Strangely enough, I don't seriously believe that the problem will last for long. Matt has been so well. God is looking after us. And we leave for Cheshire tomorrow.

I'm wrong. As time goes on, his condition is compounded by fatigue. At one in the morning, Don wraps him in his blue dressing-gown and his blanket, and leaves for the hospital. I still don't take it too seriously, remembering back to a night in January when we had gone through a similar drill. Matt had spent the night at Children's Hospital, but had been back home next morning, none the worse for wear.

It's 4 a.m. The bedroom door opens. Don shakes me from a fitful sleep. His eyes look wild. He's distraught and bewildered. He doesn't know what to do. Matthew is labouring now, barely able to take in enough air to live, and totally exhausted. Don tells me that I.C.U. is chaotic. Although Matt has been admitted, no one seems to be too disturbed by his condition. This isn't hard to understand — Matthew has been running and playing around P.S.U. all week. This is the child who joked and laughed and teased, the one who didn't even look ill.

I'm dressed in minutes and out in the parking lot. The night is pitch-black. Thank God for Brenda's car.

Don wasn't exaggerating; Matthew is literally fighting for every breath. He sits on the edge of the bed, leaning over a table. It's the best position for him, but it's still not working. He's forced to strain at each gasping inhalation. He knows I'm there, but hardly responds. I wet a cloth and cool his brow. I rearrange the pillow he leans on. They're merely token gestures, band-aids. We've lost control again.

"Where are you, God?" I shriek silently into the night. "How can you stand by and let a child suffer? I thought you promised to help us! We didn't come this far only to have him die now."

Matthew's room is across from I.C.U. I leave him struggling, and, hiding anger and distress, approach a nurse standing close to the door.

"Matthew seems to be getting worse," I tell her. "Can we do something for him?" The nurse is young and attractive, her blond hair pinned up at the back of her head.

"Dr. Jensen has already seen him," she says gently. "I'll ring him again." Dr. Jensen arrives at Matt's bedside a few minutes later. He injects Lasix into a leg muscle.

"I'm hoping it will take some fluid off his lungs," he explains kindly. "It'll make him pass water. Does he have a urinal handy?"

The Lasix fails to ease his breathing, and the nightmare continues into the dawn and beyond. The day shift start arriving shortly after 7 a.m. Fresh-faced nurses pour into the office for report. The four weary night staff hand over their patients, anxious, no doubt, for breakfast and a good sleep. Shortly after eight, Dr. Stevens appears at the bedside. Any hope that Matt will recover spontaneously has disappeared. Anyone can see he's fighting for his life. Dr. Stevens is blunt, confident, decisive. A brief examination tells him all he needs to know. He disappears and returns quickly with more Lasix, which he injects into a vein. A nurse comes to help, and together they put in an arterial line.

"Now we can keep a check on his blood gases," he explains abruptly. I'm glad to see Matt protest the procedure — there's obviously some fight there yet.

"I want to talk to you in the office," Dr. Stevens tells me. I hate talks in offices, but follow meekly. Dr. Stevens doesn't beat around the bush.

"Matthew is seriously ill," he starts. "Something critical has happened in his disease process, and he could go either way. As you know his assessment for a transplant isn't completed yet. A decision can't be made without a CAT scan. Unless he improves soon, it may be necessary to ventilate him."

"But we don't want him on a respirator unless he can have a transplant," I protest, scarcely able to grasp the change in our fortunes. "We don't want to prolong this unless there's a chance he'll be well again."

"I know, I know." Dr. Stevens is equally frustrated. "We'll monitor him carefully and see how he goes."

I return to Matt's room, numb and heartbroken. This wasn't meant to happen. It wasn't in the plan. To my immense relief, Matt seems quieter now. The gasping is over. He's more restful, more peaceful. Could it be that the Lasix is working? That the crisis was temporary, and is almost over?

I'm drained and exhausted. I need to escape and cry away the aching pain inside my chest. It occurs to me that there is nothing on earth as monstrous as this — to watch your child suffer, slip toward death, and be unable to help or to change the course. At what point, I wonder, would insanity set in? At what point would the immune system, succumbing to the excruciating stress, plant the seeds of illness and disease?

It's almost noon when, with Matt sleeping peacefully, I leave the hospital. Mrs. King is in the kitchen. Her white face searches mine, but I have little to offer by way of solace. Don is still sleeping. I hate to wake him — to bring him back to our reality.

"Shift change, hon," I whisper, shaking him gently. The phone rings, and a minute later, Mrs. King is calling up the stairs.

"Mrs. Ekroth. It's P.S.U."

"Oh no! What now?" I groan, running to the door. Don is out of bed and pulling on his clothes before I leave the room. I don't catch the Sister's name, just fragments of what she is saying. When I piece them together, I have the picture. Matt was unrousable. His respirations had dropped to a dangerous level. The respiratory team was called. He's now being taken to I.C.U. Would we come at once.

"Everything all right?" Mrs. King asks.

There's no time to weep or wonder why, no time to rave or agonize. But guilt and failure — I cannot keep them at bay. I left him when he needed me most. He was unconscious before my very eyes. "Sleeping peacefully," I had told Mrs. King. He was heading into respiratory arrest. How had I missed that? I'm a nurse as well as his mother. He might have died . . . while I was sipping coffee and preparing for sleep, he might have died . . .

"Come on in. He's awake now and asking for you." We don't know this nursing Sister. She's tall and slim, with dark curly hair and enormous blue eyes.

"Matthew, your mum and dad are here now. There's a boy." Matt is propped up in a bed by the window. He looks pale and tired, but to my relief he's no longer struggling for breath.

"You're looking better now, son," Don tells him, taking one of the small hands in his own.

"That was a pretty miserable night, guy," I add, reaching to hold the other hand.

"What?" Matt screws his face up uncomprehendingly. "You know," Don continues. "Last night, when you were having trouble breathing? It sure was no fun. Right?" Matt looks puzzled, but says nothing.

"Don't you remember, Matt?" I ask, delighted at the possibility. He shakes his head, apparently oblivious to the whole nightmare.

"Well, that's the good news!" Don whispers over his head.

"I could cope with a touch of amnesia myself," I murmur back.

The pretty nurse returns to the end of the bed.

"Matthew will probably want to sleep now," she says. "He's very tired. Have you had any lunch yet? Well, maybe you'd like to do that, then?" I'm hesitant. The last time I left, Matt almost died.

"Matthew will be fine," the Sister adds, as though reading my mind. "He'll have his own nurse all the time in here."

The local pub's white wine is tepid and too sweet. We gulp it down regardless, longing for its medicinal effects. The pain doesn't leave, but it is dulled, and can now at least be tolerated.

"We must phone my mum, hon. 'She'll be expecting us this evening. She's going out right now stocking up on food. Bet there's not an inch of space in her kitchen without a tin of something on it!"

We're miserably disappointed, too.

"What's it to you, God?" I think bitterly. "Is it too much to ask to keep him well till the operation?"

As expected, Mum is distressed, and anxious to hear of the latest developments. And yes, also as expected, she did "nip out" and "get in a little food, dear." I can well imagine!

"We'll phone you tomorrow, Mum," Don tells her. "Who knows, maybe it was an isolated episode. Perhaps we can make it up to Cheshire in a few days."

Dr. Jensen is talking to Sister at the door of I.C.U. He reminds me of my brother — the same gentleness, the same calm acceptance of life's adversities.

"Can I talk to you a minute?" Sister moves on, pushing a drug-trolley in front of her. "We've contacted Mr. Murad," he tells us. "He feels it's vital that we complete Matt's assessment as soon as possible. We don't have a scanner here. We have to use the one at Mt. Vernon Hospital. His CAT scan is booked for four this afternoon. I'll be travelling with him. I'm sure you'd like to come too?"

It's a pleasant ten-minute ride through country lanes over to the hospital. Matthew is feeling better, and quite enjoys his ride on a stretcher. He even tries a little kidding with the ambulance men. There is just one problem: the scanner has broken down. We wait for nearly an hour, hoping the problem can be solved, but in the end, we have to return to Harefield with our mission thwarted.

We see Matt settled for the evening, and, exhausted ourselves, kiss him goodnight before heading back to our haven at Sanctuary Close. Mrs. King has obviously been out somewhere special. She's wearing a smart outfit with high-heeled shoes and a matching hat. She has made up her face, but it doesn't disguise her sadness.

"I saw him," she tells us. "I walked along outside I.C.U. and peeked in the window. I had to see him for myself." Her eyes glisten and she blows her nose loudly. Dear Mrs. King — our support is coming from unexpected quarters.

It's 8 p.m. when we each down a sleeping pill. They're only a mild, over-the-counter brand, but necessary for days such as this.

"Cheers." We clank our water glasses together in mock celebration. We must look a sight: two white faces, with matching red-rimmed eyes and swollen lids. Don is writing in his journal. I'm puttering as I often do before bed — dabbing at eye make-up, cleaning teeth — comforting, routine things. The phone rings downstairs. The kitchen door opens, as we knew it would, and Mrs. King calls up the stairs.

"Mrs. Ekroth or Mr. Ekroth! It's P.S.U." Don pulls his dressing-gown around him and, with apparent casualness, descends to the kitchen below. He returns a few minutes later — no panic, no rush. "They're having a few problems with his breathing again. They'd like us to come over and make some decisions for the night." Don speaks slower than usual. His eyes are distinctly glassy.

"You look how I feel," I tell him ruefully. The sleeping pills are hard at work, dulling our senses and sapping the last of our strength. Fifteen minutes later, we're dressed, organized and ready to leave. The phone rings again. I answer it in the hall. The voice at the other end is taut and anxious. It wants to know if we're coming right away. Decisions, it tells me, must be made immediately. I stammer apologies. We hadn't, I explain, understood that it was urgent. I promise that we'll be there in a few minutes. But the voice has already gone. We're running across the parking lot, numbed with fear and medication.

"You didn't tell me it was urgent," I turn on Don. "I didn't think it was," he retorts. But I know what has happened, for we have both been guilty of this manoeuvre on occasion. Don could stand no more today. He had interpreted the information to suit his ability to cope. He simply couldn't handle another crisis.

We run like two drunks from the hospital parking lot, down the corridor, and into P.S.U. Dr. Stevens stands by the office door. He's brief and to the point. He tells us that Matt's blood gases are dangerously abnormal, and his condition is deteriorating. His opinion is that Matt will die in the next few hours if there is no intervention. The respiratory team anaesthetist has recommended immediate ventilation. The main dilemma, he reminds us, is that the assessment is not complete. There is no guarantee of a transplant.

Don's eyes are manic, something like those of a trapped animal. I suspect that mine look much the same. Stunned and speechless, all we can do is look at each other in horror. Fortunately, Dr. Stevens is not short of an opinion.

"I feel we have no option but to ventilate him," he continues. "Maybe, once he's had a good rest, he'll be able to manage on his own again. But until Mr. Murad can make a decision, we should give him every chance available." The interview over, Dr. Stevens hurries from the office and toward I.C.U. Another Sister, whose name is Karen, leads us down to the parents' lounge.

The tall, handsome man, who has kept vigil all week with the baby, sits on the sofa, his arm around an attractive dark-haired woman. They speak intently, a language we don't understand, to another man of similar age. Don and I sink into two remaining armchairs. We are dozy, incredulous and battered. The second man turns to Don and speaks in broken English. Using mime, guesswork, and a small Italian/English dictionary, they exchange stories. The threesome, we learn, are from Palermo in Sicily. Giampiero is cousin to the baby's father, Giuseppe. Baby Lorenzo was born with a serious heart condition. He needs a risky operation to give him any chance to live. Giuseppe had brought Lorenzo to Harefield immediately and Giampiero had followed a few days later, after seeing to business commitments. Luciana has just arrived, having needed a few extra days to recover from the birth. There is much in the way of drama throughout the recital — much clutching at his heart, counting on his fingers, shaking of his head, not to mention the necessary thumbing through the dictionary. Don, in turn, relates our story in a similar fashion. Every few sentences, Giampiero turns to the others and interprets the saga into their language.

Luciana catches my eye. We don't need a common language to share our fears.

Sister Karen appears at the door. "You can come and see Matthew now," she says kindly, waiting for us to join her. We rise as one, and nod goodbye to our new friends.

"He's had some drugs to put him out, so he'll not wake up for you," she warns us in her gentle way. "The tube to the respirator is in one nostril. It's taped in place, so he's got tape across his face. All right?" She speaks slowly, allowing us time to absorb the changes we must now accept. All right! Our six-year-old is breathing by grace of an electrical machine. How could it possibly be all right?

"Yes, fine, thank you," I say.

But we needn't have been so scared. Yes, there's a tube in his nose, and a large metal box purring at the head of his bed. Yes, there's a cardiac monitor, and leads sprawling across his chest. And yes, an intravenous line into his arm feeds him now that he can't feed himself. But in spite of it all, something wonderful has happened. For the first time in a year, he can lie on his back. Flat on his back. Not propped up, or hunched over a table. But flat, normal, like other children. His eyes are closed, his face serene.

A woman in operating-room greens stands by the bed. She watches Matt closely, then shifts her gaze to the softly purring machine.

"This is Dr. Travis, the anaesthetist," Sister Karen makes the introductions. Dr. Travis turns and smiles warmly in our direction.

"This is Matthew's dad and mum," Sister Karen tells her needlessly, before hurrying away to answer the phone. For the second time in as many minutes, we're informed about Matthew's support apparatus.

"Everything is working well," the doctor tells us cheerfully. "Matthew's vital signs are good. We'll see how he is tomorrow, and maybe take him off the respirator." She exudes confidence, born, I assume, of many years of experience. When we leave Matthew's side a few minutes later, we have a new perspective once more — and the all-important hope.

We're halfway down the corridor when we're stopped in our tracks. There's an urgency to Sister Karen's call. She runs from the nurses' office to where we stand. We're rooted to the spot, filled with dread at the thought of any further distressing news.

"Mr. Murad is here," she says, laying a hand on my arm. "He'd like to have a talk with you." She guides us back to the nurses' office. I feel sick and dizzy. What if he says no? What if it can't be done? Our hope may end with this interview. How will we tell Matthew? How will we prepare for his death? Prepare both him and ourselves? Say yes, Mr. Murad. Please say yes.

The tall, commanding figure of Hiram Murad stands in the doorway facing into the room. He wears the same dark-blue suit, and studies an X-ray which he holds up to the light.

"These are Matthew's parents, Mr. Murad," Sister Karen interrupts. The eminent surgeon turns, and extends a hand in greeting. His face is gentle and calm. He exudes an aura of intelligent confidence — charisma is probably the best word to describe it. I try not to grovel, not to plead — with practice, we've become good actors.

Mr. Murad outlines the situation as he sees it. No words are wasted, no emotion expended. Matthew, he says, is a high-risk patient. His disease is virtually unknown. There are other factors to consider. Major nerves might possibly be damaged. The surgery may be impossible, and even if attempted, haemorrhage is bound to be an enormous problem. Also, he points out, we still have no CAT scan pictures. He is sorry, he tells us, but a decision cannot be made without them.

With heavy hearts, Don and I return to Mrs. King's, and escape into a drugged sleep.

We awake at nine the next morning, feeling human once more. Don phones P.S.U. Matthew, the Sister tells him, was stable throughout the night. He and an anaesthetist have gone by ambulance to Wembley Hospital, where the all-important CAT scan will be done. She also tells Don that Mr. Murad has sent to the Mayo Clinic for Matt's previous CAT scan results. "They'll probably be another hour or so," she says. "We'll soon know what's what."

We enjoy a leisurely breakfast with Mrs. King, and prepare for another day.

It's mid-morning when we amble into the hospital. Dr. Travis is again standing by Matt's bed.

"Good morning," she calls gaily. "Matthew has just come off the respirator. He's doing fine, aren't you, Matthew? Look who's come to see you!" She moves aside, so Don and I can crowd around him, one on each side of the bed. We each hold a small bony hand in one of ours and caress his head or shoulder with the other. Our actions are symbolic: we yearn to protect our child. I want to pick him up and hug him to me, to keep him free from pain and harm. But if we've learned one lesson, it's this: we're impotent and powerless. We cannot protect him.

Matt is sleepy and spaced-out.

"Just rest, Matt," I tell him, "you've had a lot of drugs, which is why you feel so strange."

"I want to cry, but I can't," he says. He shuts his eyes tightly in an attempt to squeeze out some tears, but without success. Don washes Matt's face and hands, gently removing dried blood and glue that have caked around his nose.

The day passes peacefully enough, with Matt able to get up and play later in the afternoon. At seven-thirty, the night staff arrive, and the other children are settling for the night. Matthew has no such intentions.

"I'm not tired, Dad," he insists, leaning over the bed for support. "I want to play with my Transformers." We finally have to order him in, but then he refuses to close his eyes.

"What if the same thing happens again?" he asks, throwing some light on his strange behaviour. "What if I can't breathe?"

"Well, let's say a prayer about it, Matt," I coax, "and then you won't be scared." He clasps his hands tightly together, and closes his drooping eyes.

"Dear God," he prays, "don't let me be afraid. Please help Mr. Murad to get me better again."

The night passes uneventfully, and the next day, Sunday, Matt feels well enough to be up and dressed.

Just before lunchtime, he's resting on his bed, and I'm reading his favourite story for the umpteenth time. He listens attentively, lost in the magic of "Puss in Boots." We all, it seems, find our means of escape, no matter how short-lived. I hear voices in the corridor. They're not speaking a foreign language. Their familiarity warms my heart, though they're strangely out of place in here.

"Mrs. Ekroth," a nurse calls through the door, "you've got some visitors." Leaving Matt to thumb through his book, I scurry to the corridor outside. There, waiting anxiously are my mother, my sister Brenda and her husband, Roy.

"Katie," Mum says, stepping forward with a hug, "we had to come and see you, and see that little fellow for ourselves." My mum is older, greyer and sadder than I remember her. But then, I muse, I'm probably older, greyer and sadder than she remembers me, too. It's nearly a year since she stayed with us in Canada — and what a year! Don joins us, gives a round of bear hugs, then hastily retreats into I.C.U. to get Matthew. We move down the corridor toward the parents' lounge, and Matt ambles out of the unit behind us.

"Hello, Granny Petal," he calls, breaking into a run of sorts. She stoops to hug him, and his thin arms wrap around her neck. He lays his soft cheek against hers and closes his eyes, savouring the moment. For Mum, the reunion is bittersweet. Matt was relatively well when she last saw him. He suffered from a "cough," "a touch of bronchitis." He was a normal little boy with a happy life ahead of him. Since then he has frequented intensive care units, weathered miserable tests, and, quite literally, fought for his life. We have quietly watched his deterioration — inch by inch, ounce by ounce. We've seen the sparkle dim in his eyes, noted the pallor of once-healthy skin. My mum hasn't had the luxury of preparation. As Matt ambles back to his bed, she buries her head in her hands and weeps for her much-loved grandson.

Roy, Bren and Mum leave at 4 p.m. for the four-hour drive back to Cheshire.

"I've never had a sadder year," Mum tells me as we hug goodbye. "Not in the war years, not even your father's death can compare to the agony of this."

"I know, Mum," I say. "I know just what you mean."

We stay with Matt until ten, then, seeing him comfortably settled, return to Mrs. King's.

When I awake the next morning our room is drenched in bright sunshine. Only the cooing of the doves breaks the silence. Don's bed is empty and unmade — a sure sign that he left in a hurry. Mrs. King is sipping coffee in the kitchen.

"Everything all right?" she asks, concerned as always. And then, before I can answer, "I heard the phone at half past six."

"I'm sure Don would have phoned if there was a problem," I tell her. But my appetite has gone, and my companion, fear, has returned once more.

I.C.U. is alive with activity, and it's centred mainly around Matt's bed. Don meets me halfway across the unit.

"He's back on a respirator," he tells me. "He couldn't breathe again."

"Why didn't you call me?" I hiss through clenched teeth. "I've been sitting drinking coffee while Matt was being ventilated. Why on earth didn't you phone?"

"I could handle it," he calmly replies, "and you needed the rest."

I leave I.C.U. rather than make a scene. I'm boiling mad — strange for me, who's usually so placid. As I walk around the grounds, my anger slowly fades, and I realize, too, that Don is neither the cause nor the object of my rage.

I return to I.C.U. Matt is sedated, but obviously not well enough. He beckons urgently as I come through the door, then, placing his hands together as though in prayer, soundlessly begs for the tube to come out. Fluids and mucus collect in the tubes, forcing him to choke for air. Trudy, his nurse, selects a clean catheter, attaches it to the suction, and inserts it into the metal tube. He gags and coughs, my precious son, fighting for air and fighting the tube as well. Dr. Stevens injects a drug into his IV line. Trudy holds one hand and I the other.

"There you are, Matt," she says. "The medicine will make you nice and sleepy, so the old machine won't bother you." Within seconds, his eyes are closed. He has mercifully escaped from the world of blood tests, doctors, and life-support machines.

The sluice, as it is called, is a large, cold room which houses the parents' washroom facilities, a clothes-washing machine, the children's bathtub, and the inevitable bedpan washer. It's not the perfect spot to stand and weep, but it has to do. Another parent, "Mrs. Egypt," sidles past us apologetically, and nods in sympathy. Don and I cling to each other, sobbing uncontrollably.

We're not mentally prepared. This wasn't part of the plan. Not only is Matthew suffering, but we still don't know if he's eligible for a transplant. The stark reality of our situation hits us both together — if Mr. Murad can't operate, then we face the nightmare of "unplugging the machine."

After what seems like hours, though it's probably only ten minutes, we shuffle out, with bowed heads, from our hideout. Dr. Stevens is in the corridor, and has been looking for us.

"I know it's upsetting for you," he says, seeing our reddened, swollen eyes, "but you should bear in mind that, because of the high level of carbon dioxide in Matthew's blood, he'll probably remember very little of that incident." We grasp the suggestion like a lifeline — he's had amnesia with terrifying episodes before. We, unfortunately, will never forget.

Dragging ourselves to the parents' lounge, we realize that we are not the only family having an anxious day. The tiny Italian baby, Lorenzo, is in the operating theatre. His waiting family nervously bombard us with mostly mimed questions as to how Matt is faring today. They form part of our support group, and we do the same for them.

Many of the parents on this ward are thousands of miles from home and from the vital support of friends and family. In this frightening and highly charged situation, people of different colours, cultures and tongues bond in friendship in record time. We need each other. We tell our friends about Matthew by means of English, French, a smattering of Italian, hand signals, and numerous facial expressions. We learn about Lorenzo in the same way. There's no news as yet. We hug them all, show them our crossed fingers, and go out for lunch.

"'Ey up — God's comin' down the corridor," Sid, one of the fathers, announces in his broad Lancashire accent. We're sitting in the parents' lounge, watching the nine o'clock news. Don doesn't stir, but I know that, like me, he's drained and heartsick and unprepared for what we may hear. A few minutes later, Sister Sarah's pretty face appears at the door.

"Mrs. Ekroth, Mr. Ekroth, Mr. Murad would like to see you. He's in the nursing office." We follow her down the corridor, silently. I dare not hope, for fear of another crashing disappointment — but neither can hope be completely relinquished. The big man stands in the office, poring over reports and X-rays. As before, he wastes no time with small talk.

"We've closely examined the CAT scan results, as well as the ones from the Mayo Clinic," he starts. "I've also talked to Dr. Pirie and Dr. Le Blanc in Vancouver. Because of previous surgery and subsequent infection, there will be the complication of scar tissue. Added to that, the haemangioma will cause excessive bleeding. It may, consequently, be very difficult to remove the lungs." The big man pauses, as though to give us time to absorb these facts. I fight to stay calm, and wonder how Don is doing behind that mask of nonchalance. He's giving us his verdict, I think, but trying to break it to us gently. I can hardly believe his next words.

". . . difficult, yes. But not impossible. Matthew should be given every chance at life. If we find a suitable donor, we will go ahead with the transplant."

"Thank you, Mr. Murad," I say, inwardly screaming with relief. Don is hopping from foot to foot. I have a terrible feeling that he is going to hug the surgeon.

"Please don't, Don," I plead silently. Mr. Murad is Egyptian. I'm sure it's not the done thing. Somehow Don succeeds in restraining himself.

"If you can get him through the surgery, he'll make it," Don says, more excited than a child on Christmas Eve. "He's a fighter. He'll give it everything he's got." I'm nodding in agreement, for it's true. Matt has always been a fighter. He'll certainly do his part — and we'll do ours.

"Thank you, Mr. Murad," we say, over and over. "Thank you."

We kiss our sleeping son goodnight, relieved beyond words that he'll get a chance — and that our precious hope is still intact.

Diane Kent visits us the next day with more good news. Ironic though it may seem, in the world of transplants there's a definite advantage to being in critical condition. Matt has automatically jumped to the top of the waiting list for organs of his lung size and blood group. Who says there are no silver linings? Diane is guarded, however, when we ask about the wait.

"Surely it can't be long," I say, "not with the huge catchment area for organs. I can't believe it will take long." But Diane won't commit herself.

"We'll see," she says quietly. "They may come tomorrow, or not for six months." Matt, of course, needs them as of yesterday. We can only hope and pray that it won't be long.

Matthew has been put on a different respirator, one that assists his own breathing rather than completely taking over. He's heavily sedated and sleeps much of the time. We take turns sitting with him, which is easy when he's asleep.

Lorenzo has survived his operation. His incubator occupies one of the four spaces in the small I.C.U. Spasmodic beeps and flashing lights from the monitors contrast sharply with the studied, efficient movements of the staff. Each child has his or her own nurse, who continually monitors and charts every vital sign and gain or loss of fluid. The ward Sister oversees them all, checking charts, graphs, drug dosages and patients themselves. She frequently updates the surgical teams and ward doctors, who descend or phone in for information at all hours. Maybe surprisingly, laughter is often heard in the unit. No doubt it lightens the load, provides a means of surviving the stress and sadness that mark many a shift. It's also obvious that seemingly carefree banter doesn't diminish the nurses' concern for their patients nor detract from the quality of care they give.

Chapter Eleven

Tuesday, July 8

There's a card in the mail today from a lady we've never met. I guess from the somewhat unsteady writing that she's elderly, or maybe infirm.

"Dear Matthew," it says, "I saw your picture in the Sunday paper, and wanted to let you know I am thinking of you. God loves you, and so do I. Get well soon. Alice Dodd."

Bidie, an old friend from nursing school days, comes to visit. Clutching a tin of cookies in one hand and her two-year-old Dan with the other, she hurries down the corridor toward us.

"Hello, old fruit," she says, just as she did twenty years ago. "How are you keeping, then? You look all right, you know!" It's been almost three years since I've seen her, but it feels like yesterday — for this is a friendship founded on stone. We had nudged and prodded each other through training, tending to wounds of the ego inflicted by bitchy ward Sisters. We had joked and laughed together, knowing the world to be our oyster, and mourned as one for lovers false and lost.

"We can't stay long today, I'm afraid — I've got to fetch Judy from pre-school. But we'll come, if we can, to see you each week."

My brother, John, arrives unexpectedly from Liverpool. Matthew blows kisses to him across the unit. Monitor lights flash, and the respirator, totally confused, shrieks in alarm!

Charlotte Grant is back on the ward again.

"She's lost her appetite, and has awful diarrhoea," Clare tells us. "They think it's because of the cyclosporine." It's little more than a month since Charlotte's transplant, and it's quite possible that the dosage needs to be reassessed.

"Just a minor hiccup, hopefully," she says in her usual sunny way.

Thursday, July 10

Clare woke up this morning to see a small mouse staring at her from a hole in the wall. Don is waylaid, enroute to Matt's bed, to deal with the intruder. It's yet another of many contrasts we've seen since coming to the hospital. Harefield, whose medical staff are on the leading edge of transplant technology; Harefield, where intricate, delicate heart operations are performed almost daily; Harefield, home to field mice that peek at patients from holes in the walls.

Matt seems almost resigned to being on the respirator. The nurses have to suction the tubes frequently. It's miserable, uncomfortable, and frightening at times. Matthew is becoming proficient at sign language and lip-reading, and he's also mastered the art of using his vocal cords in a limited fashion. When all else fails, he'll often "talk" in spite of the tube. When I'm with him, I somehow feel redundant. I know it's mainly frustration and guilt at how little I can really do to help.

Baby Lorenzo is critically ill tonight. His heart rate is high and his blood pressure alarmingly low. His temperature is 104 degrees Fahrenheit. His parents and cousin huddle together in the corridor and shake their heads silently in response to our unspoken question. Doctors from the surgical team have been called to I.C.U. No one is smiling.

Friday, July 11

We were awakened by the helicopter again last night.

Don leaves Mrs. King's at eight in the morning. An hour later, when I join him at the hospital, it's obvious that he's been crying.

"It's Lorenzo," he whispers, as I bend to kiss our son. One glance at the incubator tells its own story. A priest is administering last rites to the tiny infant. I stare in disbelief at the monitors — the need for clergy is obvious. Giuseppe and Luciana stand close by, holding each other and weeping. Giampiero waits in the corridor.

"The doctors can't do any more," Don says. "There're no more drugs to give." Lorenzo hovers between life and death. All we can do is pray.

The O.R. has been working to capacity, Don tells me. Not only was a heart/lung transplant performed last night, but another is in progress now. We are greatly encouraged. Please God, let there be organs soon.

Lorenzo fights to live all day. By evening, miraculously, he is slightly improved.

Matthew has a fever tonight. He must be as strong as possible to survive the transplant, so any complication is threatening. Antibiotics are started to fight off any infection.

By 10 p.m. Don and I are weary, and looking forward to bed. Gayle is Matt's night nurse. She's one of his favourites, and an excellent nurse to boot, so we know he's in good hands. We help her settle him down for the night, washing his hands and face and rubbing his back. Suddenly, without any warning, Matt goes into a paroxysm of coughing. His face is puce; his eyes crazed. It's obvious that the tube is blocked.

"All right, Matt. We'll just get some suction." Gayle quickly reaches for the tubing at her side. I'm suddenly aware that Matt is urinating. It comes in a strong and steady stream, wetting and staining the bottom sheet. I'm temporarily mesmerized — this child is nearly seven, after all — but one look at his face shocks me out of my inertia. His eyes are slowly rolling back. He's stopped breathing.

I've worked both in emergency rooms and on resuscitation teams. There's a strict procedure to follow in cases of arrest. Running to the middle of the room, I yell, "Code! Code! Code! Code!" Strangely, I can hear no sound, but I know from the activity that ensues that others have heard. Peter, a senior nurse who is caring for Lorenzo tonight, rushes to the phone to put out the crash call. "Leave," I tell Don, as one would to a parent. He's almost in shock, and seems riveted to his spot by the bed. "Go away," I repeat, and stuporously he obeys. Gayle continues suctioning the tubes, and Peter has started cardiac massage. Sister Sarah appears. I stand at the head of the bed talking to Matt and kissing his cheek. "Can I stay?" I plead, knowing that really she should send me away. She nods assent, then turns to some of the resuscitation team who have spilled through the doorway and are assessing the situation.

Within seconds, the room is filled with people — some doctors, some nurses — mainly in operating greens. A few minutes later, Don and I are in our usual spot in the sluice room. We hold each other, tears streaming, sobbing uncontrollably. "That was a close one," I say.

The anaesthetist is still at Matt's bed when we return. "We caught him very quickly," he comforts. "According to the nurse, his heart rate never dropped below 40. We believe that no serious damage has been done. He'll remember little or nothing about what has happened — he has not suffered unduly. Try to believe that."

Saturday, July 12

Matthew is quite put out by our having slept in this morning. The irony almost makes me laugh — I'm so pleased to see the spark of anger in his eyes. To our considerable relief, he doesn't seem to remember the events of the previous night. Don gives him a fierce hug, and I plant kisses on his head. His wrath is defused at once.

Don badly needs some summer shirts, and we want to buy soft towels for Matt. After lunch, we drive into Uxbridge and head for Marks and Spencers. The parking lot is full, the entrance a bottleneck. Droves of brightly dressed people, ambling slowly, spill from the sidewalks, blocking the streets. Nobody seems to care. Nobody, that is, but the motorists.

"Let's make this fast," I say, as we shuffle along with the crowds of shoppers, "I hate this place."

Leaving Don looking at shirts, I head toward the towels. Nothing but the best for Matt, of course. Selecting the plushest yellow set that I can find, I pay the cashier, then head back the way I came. I notice the man right away. He's lurking in the jackets and gazing intently in the direction of the shirts. He's obviously a store detective, I think, grateful for any diversion. Fascinated, I follow his gaze. It falls on the naked back of a tall, greying man who's trying on some shirts. The man in the jackets isn't the only spectator; several women have paused to observe this unusual sight in their local Marks and Spencers!

"You can't strip here, Don," I say, rushing to the offender's side. "There's a store detective watching!" But Don doesn't care. He's not, he tells me, wasting time running back and forth to Uxbridge while Matt's in I.C.U. "If Marks can't put in changing rooms, it's their own fault!" He finally chooses two shirts, pays the cashier, and we leave in haste. The store detective watches us go.

Lorenzo, miraculously, is better today. He's not out of the woods yet by any means, but his family are smiling again.

Sunday, July 13

Joan comes to visit. We'd love to find a traditional roast beef dinner. It's not to be, however. The Long Beach Restaurant in Rickmansworth is highly Americanized —roast beef is not on the menu.

Another week and still no organs. Please God, don't let it be long.

We tiptoe into the unit to say goodnight. Matt is peaceful and pink as he drops off to sleep. If we can't have the transplant now, we'll gladly settle for peaceful and pink!

Monday, July 14

As we're leaving the unit tonight, Barbara Turner, the night Sister, stops us. "I'm wondering what you've told him," she says kindly. "He's asking if he's going to die." I tell her that he asks us too. "He knows that he would have died had we still been in Canada. He's very aware that the transplant is the only chance he has."

But that, Barbara tells me, is not quite what she meant. "I was wondering about his concept of death, and whether perhaps you have a religious background? If we know these things we can reinforce what you have told him, and help to allay some of his fears."

We return to Mrs. King's, safe in the knowledge that when he asks again, Barbara will reassure him of God's promise of heaven.

Wednesday, July 16

A telegram arrives from Expo '86. "We're all hoping you get well soon, Matthew," it says. He doesn't recognize all the signatures, of course — but he's thrilled with the ones he knows.

"It's a letter from Mickey Mouse," he mouths, proudly showing the paper around.

I wander into the parents' lounge, glad for a change of scene. Two new parents are nervously watching "Coronation Street." Hilda Ogden is yapping away as only Hilda can. It's then that I notice she has competition. Mr Muhammad, the Egyptian, is kneeling on the floor of the extension, eyes shut, head bowed. He holds a book in his hands, and chants in his own language. I join the nervous twosome, and pretend that this is normal. I have to admit, the Koran and Hilda do not blend easily.

Friday, July 18

The weather has been very strange indeed. We arrived in a heat wave, and for nearly ten days it's been unbearably hot. Don finally succumbs and wears newly acquired shorts over to the hospital. By 11 a.m. the clear blue skies have clouded over and the temperature has dropped to what feels like near-freezing. "Brass monkey weather today," chortles one of the nurses, looking at Don's goose pimples.

There's a fresh patch of blood on Matt's pillow today; just one more indication of the fine line he's treading.

Charlotte is visibly better every day we see her. Ringing her bell frantically, she scoots past us on her tricycle. She's also able to play on the swings outside the unit. We know that Charlotte waited two months for a donor. Not only was she unlucky enough to have an uncommon blood type, but there was another, more critical child with the same rare type on the list ahead of her. Since Matt has a fairly common blood type, B positive, and because he's at the top of the list, we're hoping that his wait won't be long. Charlotte's presence is a big boost to our morale.

Saturday, July 19

My sister Ruth is visiting. She waves at Matt from the doorway of I.C.U. "Nice to see you," he mouths in response. It's warm and sunny again, a lazy kind of day. We lounge in lawn chairs on the patio, enjoying the break from our world of fear and illness. Visits from family and friends are a pleasant reminder that there's a whole other world out there. The sun's warm rays caress our weary bodies, relaxing our tensions and seducing us with long-forgotten memories of well-being. I close my eyes and imagine myself back home, sitting in the back yard. Bees hover around the hanging baskets, and birds visit noisily in the alder tree.

I'm aware of Don getting out of his chair on several occasions to check on Matt through the I.C.U. window. Matt is stable today, resting peacefully.

The morning passes pleasantly. Don and Ruth are engaged in conversation — nothing too serious, mainly bantering to match our mood. I rise sleepily from my chair and amble to the window. It's almost time for lunch. One last check and we'll head for the village . . . I can't believe my eyes: Matthew has arrested! Abbie is bagging him urgently. Another nurse is massaging his heart. Abbie looks up and sees my shocked, incredulous face at the window.

"Go away, Katie," she yells protectively, "we'll talk in a minute. Go away." I turn from the window in a daze. Don's laughing loudly at one of Ruth's stories. I hate to spoil this rare good time. I wish I could protect him. But already it's too late. He's seen my face, and has jumped to his feet.

Sunday, July 20

Yesterday's "hiccup" has left us tired and despondent. Fortunately, Matt was caught in time, and the offending blockage was dealt with quickly. It's obvious, however, that time is running out. Please God, let there be organs soon.

We're saved our weekly "hunt the roast beef dinner" escapade by a timely invitation from Rick and Kathy Gibbons. Rick is a Canadian news correspondent living near London. He travels much within the U.K., gleaning news for the use of the Canadian media. Rick had phoned originally to request an interview about Matthew. From there, he and Kathy had befriended us, as both fellow Canadians and fellow parents.

The chicken supper is delicious; the change in environment a tonic. Much of the conversation centres around the upcoming wedding of Prince Andrew and Sarah Ferguson on Wednesday. England has been buzzing with it for weeks now. Rick will be covering the wedding, of course. He even has a seat reserved in Westminster Abbey, but prefers to stay outside and report on the wedding as it progresses. This job definitely has some benefits!

Monday, July 21

It's our tenth wedding anniversary. There's only one present we want, of course. Hoping for this to happen, however, is at times accompanied by an overwhelming sense of guilt. For our prayers to be answered, someone else's child must die.

The ever-practical Mrs. King points out the flaw in our thinking.

"You aren't hoping for some child to die so that Matthew can live," she says. "Accidents happen every day. It's a fact of life. The tragedy is that most of these people, children and adults alike, are buried or cremated, taking good organs with them. What you're hoping for is a gift of these organs. You can't feel guilty about that — you'll drive yourselves crazy!"

We know she's right, but it still remains a highly sensitive issue.

Wednesday, July 23

The Royal Wedding Day.

Don and I are in the unit by half past nine. Matt is sedated but propped up in bed, "watching" a television. TVs are scarce in Harefield, and the nurses needed an eligible patient to sit in front of the screen! Neither baby Lorenzo nor Leah, the little Egyptian child, is a suitable candidate. Matt is as good as it gets!

We pull up chairs and sit by the bed. I hold his small bony hand in mine, and whenever he stirs, tell him about the wedding and the colourful people involved. There's a holiday atmosphere. No one complains when the nurse stops to glimpse the handsome couple. Every member of the royal family is scrutinized, and opinions are offered on each one's choice of dress. Needless to say, Princess Di's polka dots don't go unremarked. The pomp and ceremony help take our minds off immediate problems — it's therapy of the best kind.

The couple are leaving Westminster Abbey. Thousands of people wave and cheer.

"Sister," a nurse's voice yells from Leah's bed. Looking up, I see the monitor numbers changing rapidly. The nurse looks frantic and yells again, this time more urgently.

We're ushered from I.C.U. as doctors arrive on the scene. . . It was good while it lasted, a memory to keep for always.

Late in the afternoon, my sister Helen arrives. For a number of reasons, she has been a reluctant guest of British Rail for most of the day.

"I don't know how I landed at Morton-in-Marsh!" she exclaims, for the third time in as many minutes. We take her out for supper in the village and, like the rest of England on this special day, talk about nothing but the Royal Wedding.

When we return, Matt is bleeding again. His nurse keeps the suction going, and we watch anxiously as bright blood courses through the tube.

"It's from your disease, Matt," I tell him. "Won't it be great when we can get rid of it all!" He nods in agreement. His courage is amazing.

By 10:30 p.m., the haemorrhage has stopped and Matt is resting. We trudge home to bed. It's been traumatic, but somehow we have shed no tears. Maybe we're becoming hardened. We know that in some ways we're lucky. Were we at home, Matt would now be dead. Here, at Harefield, at least he has a chance — but it's getting smaller with every crisis. Please God, let there be some organs soon. Can't you see we're running out of time?

Friday, July 25

A set of organs has become available overnight. They're healthy, and exactly Matthew's size. Sadly, however, they're not the right blood group. A six-year-old French girl, Cosette, has arrived with her mother, and is in the O.R. now. Yes, I'm envious. Yes, I wish it were Matt. But there's no point wasting energy when it won't change a thing.

As we're leaving for supper, Cosette is wheeled out of surgery. Her new heart and lungs are functioning well. Her colour is good. She tells her mum she'd like some pop. Her mother, a young dark-haired woman, beams proudly, her anxiety melting even as we watch.

"Matthew soon!" she says excitedly, waving crossed fingers in the air. The sight of the child faring so well buoys our spirits immensely. For today, anyway, lunch is a happy affair.

On our return from the village, Trudy, Matt's day nurse, pulls Don aside.

"I need a little help," she says hesitantly. "Matthew's bladder is distended and he needs to be catheterized. I want to explain the procedure to him before the doctor starts, so I'm wondering what you normally call *it*." Trudy winks at Don to emphasize the "it", but despite her boldness she's a bright shade of pink.

"Oh," Don replies easily, "we always call it the real thing." (We had never subscribed to the baby-talk words like weenie, winkie, and pinkie.)

A few minutes later, Trudy returns with the catheter tray. She pulls the screens around Matt's bed.

"Just try and relax, Matt," we hear her say. "I'm just going to slide this tube into your real thing!"

We talk to Diane again today. She, like us, is frustrated. An Italian boy's heart has become available. The child is Matthew's age and his blood group is the same. Enquiries have been made about the lungs, which are both healthy and in good condition. But Italy will not release them. It's against the law, they say. They plan to change the law because of surgical progress, but for the moment, they're unable to release the lungs.

"We've been to the top," Diane tells us, "but nothing can be done." She shakes her head, she's tired today. Her job isn't all roses by any means.

There's another setback too. A number of British papers have been publishing articles dealing with the controversial elements of transplantation. The issue, it seems, is brain death — an issue which, being fundamental, has challenged medical ethics committees since the program's earliest days. In spite of the establishment of strict criteria that must be met before organ donation can occur, the ethical dilemma hasn't gone away — and it's back now, down from the shelf, ready for another examination. A few medical dissenters from the other major transplant centre, Papworth Hospital in Cambridge, are airing their doubts publicly, and anything negative is being gleefully dissected by the press.

"Organs Plucked from Live Bodies," shrieks one tabloid's headline. Another article implies that the hapless donor may "feel" the organs being removed. The more irresponsible, sensationalist members of the press are having a field day. People will die because of it, maybe people like Matthew.

Mr. Murad is in the unit tonight. He's sorry that things are moving so slowly. He's sorry that there are still no organs. We're sorry too. Everyone's sorry.

Saturday, July 26

A stable day without a crisis! Wonderful! Matt still has a chest infection, but his X-rays are clearer this morning. His nurse moves the IV needle to a vein in his groin area. His hands and arms are bruised, and badly in need of a rest. The change unexpectedly boosts Matt's morale, and he acts accordingly. With his arms free for the first time in a month, he can give us lots of hugs, and does so. He can also play with his Transformers without setting off an IV alarm. Among hills made by sheet-clad bony knees, Optimus Prime and his robot troops conduct their good-versus-evil wars.

I phone Mum to tell her that Matt's stable again. She's overjoyed, of course — and she has some heartening news for us. Helen and John have contacted several children's hospitals in the north and midlands, just to remind them of the need for organs. Helen has also written to Esther Rantzen, the popular hostess of "That's Life." She's been instrumental before, through her program, in locating organs for transplantation. Anything and everything is worth a try.

We're watching the early edition of the news. The main story is about a train crash somewhere in the north of England. A number of people have died, some of them children. I don't meet Don's gaze. Hope and guilt entwine once more.

Sunday, July 27

Still no organs today. . . .

I'm sitting by Matt's bed, reading him a story. I'm halfway through "The Happy Prince" when I feel his hand on my arm. His big blue eyes are intent and serious. He mouths four words.

"I want some . . ."

"I can't make ou the last word, Matt," I tell him. "Try again." It takes three tries before I interpret his wish. A sharp, deep sadness invades my being and the need to weep almost overwhelms me.

We often talk, this child and I, about life and death and illness, about courage and love — and about a world which is not altogether fair.

"I know, son, that you want some peace," I say, laying the book aside. "I know you want to be better, and that's what we're hoping for. You do know that it's nothing you've done or thought that's made you ill? And you do know that we all love you? It's just . . ."

Matthew grabs my arm. He shakes his head emphatically. "No! I said 'I want some pizza!'" he mouths. "Pee-eet-za!" . . . What a relief to feel like a fool!

We again eat lunch at The Tandoori in the village. Their food is very good — but no, they don't serve roast beef.

Monday, July 28

There's a new presence in the house. An elderly man from Spain now occupies Mrs. King's bedroom, while his wife and son stay a few houses away. Mrs. King has been relegated to sleeping on the couch in the living room. Jose, the man's twenty-two-year-old son, is waiting for a heart/lung transplant too. I must admit that our noses are a little out of joint. Mrs. King's has been a haven for us, a hint of a different world from the one we inhabit at I.C.U. Mr. Montez speaks no English, so breakfast, once a relaxing time of day, now becomes an extension of life in the hospital, with its sign language, pointing and desperate gesticulations.

Matthew is faring much better. He needs less sedation, which enables him to be more animated. We read books and stories to help pass the time, and now that his hands are free, he can also play card games. He and Don play many different games, but Fish is Matt's favourite. He seems to almost sense the cards, and Don doesn't have to let him win. In fact, he hardly gets a look in! Matt's eyes sparkle with delight as he forms the words "Fish upon my wish." Don groans loudly, and shakes his head in disbelief.

"OK. One more game. This time for da gran' championship o' da woild," Don drawls in his best Archie Bunker accent. Matt chalks up another victory.

"All right," Don urges. "Time for your exercises. Mrs. Merry won't be pleased if you don't do your Highland dance practice." Lying in bed, Matt does leg-ups and toe-points, as we attempt to keep his ever-shrinking muscles in some semblance of condition. Even attached to all the wires and hoses, he manages a few shaky deep knee bends beside his bed. His morale is remarkable considering he's now been on the respirator for nearly a month. Thank God for his courage and spirit.

Cosette, the French child, is up and walking, eating regular meals, and this afternoon is riding a tricycle down the corridor. Playing the game, Don leaps for safety, and she laughs and laughs. It's incredible to think that this laughing child had her operation just five days ago! We tell Matthew about her, of course. Anything positive, anything hopeful, anything that might fortify his own will to fight is passed on to him. Mr. Murad and his team can only do so much. After that it's up to us. Our attitude, our faith could mean the difference between his making it or not.

When we leave Matt, he's grinning from ear to ear, having just beaten Don at cards yet again.

Wednesday, July 30

A letter in the mail from Joy reminds us that we are far from alone.

"There was a big fund-raiser for Matthew over the weekend," she writes. "The Lion's Club and Safeway put it on. They had hot dogs and Pepsi by donation — it went very well. The Tsawwassen Business Association is helping out too. They're planning for local children to decorate tin cans this coming Saturday. I think they're going to put them in the shops, and collect money for Matthew that way." I read the letter to Matt. Like me, he seems at a loss to find the right words. Joy has enclosed a photo of Stephanie, her daughter, who is one of Matt's special friends. At barely four years of age, she is helping out as well. The picture shows her sitting behind a table at the foot of their driveway, partially hidden by an enormous jug. "Fruit Punch 25 Cents," reads the notice. "Proceeds to Matthew Ekroth Transplant Fund."

Thursday, July 31

I should have known it couldn't last. Matt's bleeding from his lungs again. This is worse than the last time. Big, fun-loving Robert is his nurse this shift. He and Matt have a special rapport. We all try to stay calm, but it isn't easy.

"Just bleeding from the disease, Matt," I tell him, seeing the fear in his eyes. "Boy, will it be nice to exchange these old duds for some good, healthy lungs!"

Jill arrives at seven for night duty. She's been up to London today and has brought back a present for Matt. Two books nestle in the bottom of a green and gold bag.

"Oh, Matt, a Harrod's bag. How wonderful! You've got a Harrod's bag!" I twitter excitedly, not entirely oblivious to the withering glance from my young Canadian son.

We leave for Mrs. King's at ten. The haemorrhage has stopped, Matt is sedated, and a blood transfusion is in progress. Goodnight, fella. Sleep well. Who knows? Maybe tomorrow . . .

Sunday, August 3

The quest for the elusive roast beef dinner begins anew. It has become an obsession, a fetish almost. Visions of Yorkshire pudding drowning in thick brown gravy, offset by fresh peas, carrots and mashed potatoes, have Don drooling as we leave the hospital parking lot. The first restaurant we try, which was recommended by one of the nurses, is closed for renovations. It's a minor setback, and our spirits remain high. The second doesn't serve Sunday lunches, and the third, only cold meals. It's twelve forty-five now and there's panic in Don's eyes. I'm conscious of the speedometer registering higher-than-normal readings.

"Slow down, Don," I snarl, "it's not that important." But Don has assumed his Sterling Moss position, and there's a slight twitch above his left eye. It's shortly after one when we screech into the parking lot of a quaint Denham pub sporting a large sign: "Sunday Special — Hot Roast Beef Dinner." Don's face softens — victory is at hand.

"Sorry, Guv," the waiter says. "We stop serving hot meals at one. Got nice pork pies today, though." Don hates pork pies. He orders two large sherries. He's very quiet. "It must be Sunday," he finally mutters.

Monday, August 4

Lorenzo is moved out of intensive care. We buy Giuseppe and Luciana a bottle of wine to celebrate. It occurs to me, not for the first time, that it seems akin to a lottery with these critically ill children who walk the fine line. . .you win . . . you lose . . . you win . . . Please God, give Matt a lucky number too.

I'm suddenly aware again of how thin he has become. In spite of the tube feeding, in spite of the IVs, in spite of the physiotherapy and exercises, his condition is considerably weaker than when we first arrived. We can't afford to wait much longer.

Tuesday, August 5

Giuseppe and Luciana invite us to lunch. With great ceremony, we set up a small table on the patio by the unit. Luciana has been to the village bakery, and has brought a selection of buns and pastries. The celebratory bottle of wine and four plastic mugs are produced with a flourish. We smile and nod, and nod and smile. We suddenly realize that we have no corkscrew, and after fruitless enquiries, Giuseppe settles for a kitchen knife.

"To Lorenzo," Don and I toast in unison. "Matthew," our hosts respond.

We bask in the sunshine, eating our buns and picking pieces of cork from our wine — and all the time, nodding and smiling.

Wednesday, August 6

Word reaches us that the young Egyptian girl is not only blind but deaf and semi-paralysed as well. No one is sure whether the conditions are permanent or temporary. Don is overwhelmed by the news. He hides behind the hospital wall, doubled up with grief.

"Leah wasn't a transplant patient, Don," I comfort, but my efforts are all in vain. Racking sobs come from his hiding-place for more than an hour. When, finally, he can talk, it is patently clear that his anguish is partly for Leah's parents and partly for ourselves.

"Do you remember what Mr. Murad told us about Matt's operation? He said the chance of serious nerve damage is quite high, because the disease surrounds not only his heart and lungs, but some major nerves too. He didn't draw pictures for us, but this is what he meant. Matt could end up blind or deaf or paralysed, or a hundred other things! Do you remember what Dr. Pirie said? That some things are worse than death? What if Matt turns into a vegetable?" Fresh tears roll down his cheeks and his body shakes with sobs once more.

I can find no words of comfort. "It's a risk we have to take, Don," I tell him. "There are no guarantees, but Matt will die for sure without the operation. We don't have a choice."

It's Robert's birthday today. It's also his last day on the unit. As a student in a postgraduate nursing course, he is moved around frequently so he can gain different experiences. Though the hospital gift shop does its best, it has a limited supply of items appropriate for male nurses in their early twenties. I settle on a colouring book, for fun, and an iced cupcake as a token for the real thing. Matt hides them both beneath his sheet, and when Robert comes to hug him goodbye, he flings back the thin cover and reveals the double surprise. The chocolate icing has melted and is smeared along two of the monitor leads. Robert accepts the gifts as if they're diamonds.

"I'll be thinking about you, Matthew," he promises. I know he means it.

Thursday, August 7

I can hardly look at Mr. and Mrs. Muhammad. We feel so bad about their misfortune. The unit is quiet. The gloom of defeat hangs in the air like a cold, rainy November morning. Despite the high success rate of the countless exceptional operations performed here, the staff seem to take the setback personally. I think of Mr. Murad and the team. What courage it must take to carry on in spite of the inevitable failures.

Matt, however, is in high spirits. I put on his favourite music, Alabama. He has a Walkman, and he beats time on his stomach. He enjoys more games of Fish with Don, and laughs and jokes with the nurses.

Saturday, August 9

Much of the morning is spent in planning our strategy for tomorrow. We drive around the local villages and eventually find what we seek in Denham. The quaint old pub is promising roast beef dinner as its Sunday special again. Laughing and relaxed, we return to Harefield. Victory is but a short car ride away.

Sunday, August 10

I decide to go to church this morning. The parish church in Harefield is tucked away down a lane off the main road to the village. It's a very old church, with graves huddled around it as if unable to be separated. The cold stone building hosts a sparse but enthusiastic congregation. There are no monitors or machines here; no tearstained faces. This is the house of God, and I feel at peace for the first time in many weeks. At the end of the service, I'm the first one to the door, with one thing on my mind. The minister is still combing his hair in preparation for the social minutes ahead. He shakes my hand warmly, and then I'm gone. Don and my sister Joan are waiting, ready to whisk me away to Denham village and the long-awaited roast beef dinner. We're there by twelve-forty. The parking lot is full.

"Oh, God. Not again," Don mutters.

"You park the car. Joan and I'll go and reserve our lunches," I tell him.

The pub is noisy, and reeks of beer and smoke. We inch our way to the bar with a sense of deja vu. The large silver meat platter is empty, save for meat juice and one fatty slice of beef. So near and yet so far. Don joins us. His language is impolite. We settle for sausage rolls and salad.

"Next week, we'll be here early," Don snarls between clenched teeth. "We're going to do it. We're going to get a roast beef dinner if it kills us!"

Monday, August 11

On arriving at the ward, I hear Don's unmistakable voice. He's reading one of the "Masters of the Universe" books that Matt particularly likes. Apart from Transformers, He-Man is the most "awesome" thing in the whole world. "You'll never take me, He-Man," snarls Skeletor, the arch-demon. Don's voice rises, and "By the power of Greyskull!" echoes throughout the unit. I'm momentarily embarrassed, but the staff just grin and go about their work. This is obviously nothing new to them.

My sister Helen and her three children arrive in midmorning. Jonathan is thirteen, Christopher is nine and Anna barely seven. Three years have passed since they last saw their Canadian cousin. One by one, they peer through Matt's window. "Hi, Matt," they say in turn.

A celebrity of sorts arrives late in the afternoon. Jamie Gavin, who one year ago was the world's youngest heart/lung transplant recipient, has arrived at Harefield for his first annual checkup. He's now four years old and the picture of health. A reporter and cameraman arrive from the BBC; Jamie is to be featured on tomorrow evening's news. He goes through his paces, somersaulting across the grass, standing on his head, sliding down the slide. His energy seems boundless. I watch from the window by Matthew's bed and describe the scene outside.

"This time last year, Jamie was waiting for his operation," I tell him. "Now he's running and jumping and laughing — pretty neat, eh?" Matthew nods his head in agreement. Suddenly, his hand grasps my arm and his eyes lock with mine. His lips mouth a question that roots me to the spot. When I don't answer him promptly, he repeats the question emphatically, and I, stalling for time, echo it aloud.

"What are we waiting for?" His face is wise for a six-year-old. His eyes do not leave mine. I bumble through my set reply.

"Well, Matt. You know. We're still waiting for Mr. Murad to be able to do the operation," but I've hardly finished the sentence when he asks the question again.

"What are we waiting for?"

Sister Karen appears like magic at the foot of the bed.

"You know, Matt," she starts, "we were talking about it this morning. Remember? We're waiting for the organs to be made. It takes time to get them just the right size. Remember now?"

I cast her a look of gratitude. I don't want to deceive our son, but I don't want to upset him either. If he weren't restricted by the respirator, we would have discussed the source of the organs a long time ago — but this isn't the right time. Matt nods his head, remembering, and the subject is dropped for the moment.

Tonight a visitor brings in an evening paper. As one of the two main London papers, it has an enormous circulation. A well-known columnist has written a scathing article on transplants. It's totally unprofessional and riddled with inaccuracies. There are flaws in the arguments that a ten-year-old could detect. The very title "Do We Really Want to Live Forever?" screams of its bias and misses the point of the transplant program entirely. Unfortunately, it's the kind of article that the average weary commuter will read and digest before moving on to the sports page. It's the kind of article that could influence people against donating organs. It's like being kicked when you're already down. I fight back tears, but am less successful with panic, rage and hatred.

"It's obvious that he's never had a child who needed a transplant," someone mutters. "I bet he'd change his tune in double-quick time then." Jean, a new mum, starts to cry.

"If they keep this up, Paul won't have a chance," she sobs. "There are very few hearts of the size that he needs as it is."

Christine, one of the staff nurses, stops by to check on the reason for our despondency. I show her the offending article, which she reads in silence. Periodically she looks up and shakes her head in disbelief.

"We're running out of time, Christine," I say quietly. Her eyes are brimming with tears.

"Yes, we're running out of time." she answers.

Tuesday, August 12

I'm writing a letter in the small parents' lounge when the hospital general manager arrives. His presence invited curiosity, as his duties rarely bring him down to P.S.U. He has met Don and me on several occasions.

"Ah, Mrs. Ekroth, there you are. I have some good news for you." The news is not merely good, it's wonderful! Apparently, my sister Helen, on returning home last night, had told her husband, David, about Jamie Gavin and the BBC news item. David, in turn, remembered that an old friend of his, James Millard, works on that very program. He called the BBC, and as chance would have it, James Millard himself is working on the story! He has offered to return to Harefield today and, using Matthew as a focus, do a story on the need for donor organs. I'm sick with nervousness, but absolutely elated at the same time. It's a chance to undo some of the damage from yesterday's newspaper. It will increase awareness again.

James Millard arrives at four, as promised, and the manager makes the introductions. The reporter begins with apologies. "This will have to be rushed, I'm afraid. We have less than two hours to get it to the studio. I can't make any promises, either. If there's a lot of high-priority news, there may not be time to add it on."

After some discussion it is agreed that Matthew can be filmed through the I.C.U. window. Everyone is very busy, but I call to Matt's nurse, "Abbie, can we wake Matt up? They want some film for tonight's news."

Matt is unhappy at being disturbed. Sleep, after all, is an escape of sorts. I plead my way into the unit, and beg him to cooperate.

"Please, Matt, this could make a difference to your getting the operation soon." He turns his head slowly and looks into the camera.

A few minutes later, after a careful briefing, the interview begins. It is short-lived. A small plane hovers overhead. It wheels and dives spasmodically — someone's having fun. It could hardly be noisier. The sound man looks up in disgust. James Millard reads the expression.

"We'll have to wait a minute," he says. The courier looks pointedly at his watch and shakes his head.

The small plane continues its manoeuvres, teasing and circling above the ground. Finally, after what seems an eternity, it sputters several times and meanders away to a new pasture. The interview takes only minutes, given the right conditions. The final words are scarcely spoken before the courier has the tape in hand. He runs for his motorbike and heads speedily into the London rush hour.

It's 6 p.m. and the parents' lounge is crowded. The newsman runs through the day's top stories, which I don't hear. Human interest features come next. Jamie Gavin peers out from the TV screen, "C'mon, ma'am. I'm tired of all this talkin'," he yells in his broad Irish accent. He slides down the slide, and stands on his head — all the things that "real" four-year-olds do. His mother, Marion, calmly talks of how ill he used to be, and of how, since the transplant, he enjoys a healthy normal life.

The scene changes abruptly.

Matthew, with all the trappings of life-support, is flashed on the screen.

"There are many children waiting for donor organs. Some will not survive the wait." The message could not be clearer. Don and I (or rather, Don's elbow and I) are shown briefly.

". . . we know it's someone else's tragedy. But it's Matthew's only chance of life."

The room erupts in excited chatter.

"It could make a difference."

"Nice shot of your elbow, Don . . ."

Several parents for whom English is still a problem bow and smile.

"Good." "Good."

Word spreads, and there's standing room only for the nine o'clock news. We perch on the edge of our seats and wait through familiar stories. The minutes tick by. What started as excitement turns to anxiety. With each new item, the audience protests.

"Oh no!"

"Come on."

"Hurry up!"

"How can they think that Mrs. Thatcher out walking her dogs is more important than children's transplants?" an indignant voice asks.

The news is over. No one is interested in the weather.

Disappointment, sharp at first — but not for long. We've had the chance to "do" something, to hold the reins for a moment. It feels so good.

Chapter Twelve

Wednesday, August 13

Another morning paper has jumped on the bandwagon.

"Organs Removed from Living Bodies," the headlines blare. Meaty. Sensational. The stuff with which tabloids are sold. We spend time composing a letter to the editor. It's all we can do. Bidie arrives at ten-thirty, carrying the now familiar tin of homemade cookies. Judy has made a card for Matt. With help from her mum, she shows it to him, leaning through the window.

Matt's out of sorts; I don't want to leave him.

"That's all right, lovey. You stay with him. That's far more important. I'll be out here with Judy and Dan."

Dr. Richmond hovers at the I.C.U. door. She glances towards me, hesitates, then disappears. Several nurses wave from the doorway. We're accustomed to friendliness and attention, but today is somehow special. I put it down to our ten-second stint on the six o'clock news, and continue with reading to Matt.

It's 11:30 a.m. Matthew's restless and grumpy. After a couple of stories, we talk about school and his friends. "I don't like being me," he mouths, "I wish I was Austen."

Dr. Richmond returns. She glances at Matt, then crosses I.C.U. and beckons me to where she stands at the foot of the bed. There's no warning, no introduction, no bugles or clashing of cymbals. Simply a whisper.

"We think we have some organs for Matthew. If so, the transplant will take place later today. I'll let you know shortly." And she's gone. ·

We're accustomed to the effects of adrenalin now. The physical changes on hearing this news are more than familiar. But this is a little different. Along with the pounding heart, the nausea, the dry mouth, the interminable fear, is a rare and joyous sense of relief. Matt will get his chance to live, after all.

Dr. Richmond returns within minutes.

"It's on," she whispers. "It's scheduled for eight o'clock tonight. Does your husband know?" I shake my head, temporarily dazed. "Would you like me to tell him?"

"Yes, please. I think he's either on the patio or in the toy room. And, Dr. Richmond, thank you."

Bidie waves through the window again, just checking that all is well.

"Well, lovey, how's it going?" she asks. I tell her, most thankful that she is here to share our special news.

"We'll go, lovey. There'll be lots going on here today." She turns to call the children. "Judy. Dan. Come on. We have to go now. Come and wave goodbye to Matthew." Matt opens his eyes and waves to the sweet, curious faces at the window.

Nurses wave and wink from the doorway. Don arrives. His face is flushed and he wears a studied expression of nonchalance. His eyes meet mine, and speak volumes. We stand at Matt's bed, one on each side, holding his hands and making some pretence at conversation. All the time we're studying the little boy, drinking in the sight of him, the colour of his eyes, the length of his dark lashes, the contour of his nose, the sweetness of his mouth. We find some pretext for leaving his bedside. There are things to be said, to be arranged. Strangely enough, it has all been said before in anticipation of this moment. The "if onlys," the "maybes," the "what ifs" — they've been rehearsed over and over.

"This is the chance we came for," Don says. "He may die on the table, but at least he will have had the chance. He's on borrowed time at the moment. We have nothing to lose, and everything to gain." We both need the affirmation.

"Let's not tell Matt till nearer the time," I suggest. "There's no point in having him worried and frightened all afternoon." Don agrees.

We return to I.C.U. Matt has fallen asleep, oblivious to the excitement surrounding him. We share our great news with the other families — Clare and Charlotte, Jamie Gavin's parents, Mr. and Mrs. Muhammad, some new parents — Mr. and Mrs. Kuwari from Uganda, Mr. and Mrs. Montez, and of course Giuseppe and Luciana. We then part company. Don heads off to phone family and friends, and I head for Mrs. King's and a long hot bath, which I suddenly can't live without!

Don returns to Matthew an hour later, only to find him surrounded by nurses, doctors and anaesthetists. Matt is bewildered, of course, by all the sudden attention, and it's obvious that an explanation is needed immediately. Don waits for a lull in the medical activity, takes a deep breath, and plunges in. We know the importance of attitude, and Don wastes no time in repeating each positive point to our frightened son. He points to the picture of Jamie Gavin, (which is taped above the bed), and reminds Matthew of Charlotte. He reminds him, too, of what the operation can accomplish, and of a possible return to former activities. Together they talk of bike rides, trips to the waterslides, fishing with rods on lazy days — and last, but certainly not least, there's the promise of that new skateboard! When I arrive on the scene, they're saying a prayer. Matt's eyes are closed tightly and his thin hands are clenched together. Don's words are for all of us. "Please may Mr. Murad be successful, and please don't let me be scared."

We have two hours to calm Matthew and answer his many questions. He's disappointed to hear that he'll still be attached to the respirator after the transplant, but we assure him that it will just be until the new lungs can work on their own. We're careful not to convey the terrible fear gnawing inside us, and fight back the urge to hold and hug him for what may be the last time.

It is a precious time indeed — each minute has worth and weight. We reassure and encourage, we touch and love. We make sure that everything we need to say is said. We help Wendy, the nurse, with his bedbath and preparation, and when the anaesthesia team arrives with the stretcher at seven-thirty, we know it has all been done. There will be no regrets.

"Be peaceful, Matt. God is looking after you," I whisper, as I gently kiss him goodbye.

The summer evening is fine and warm and, in spite of its being a Wednesday, the Orchard Restaurant is as busy as on many weekends.

"About an hour's wait, sir," the waitress tells Don. That's fine with us. We have nothing planned for the evening anyway. We take our glasses of wine to one of the wooden tables outside and drink in the sights and sounds around us.

At the next table, a couple talk and flirt in the intimate way reserved for lovers. Behind us is a group of young men in their early twenties. Raucous laughter emanates from their beer-strewn table, testimony to the fact that the "boys" are out on the town. From inside the restaurant, the clatter of plates and the murmur of table conversations drift across the warm evening air. It's all so normal.

We raise our glasses in a silent toast.

By eleven we're back at the hospital. Dr. Richmond meets us in the corridor. She tells us that Mr. Murad is using special laser equipment to remove Matt's lungs. The retrieval team should be arriving with the donor organs within a couple of hours. The news is good so far, and that's all we have to deal with.

Back on P.S.U., the night staff greet us excitedly. The housekeeping team have already been in and scrubbed the walls and floor of the transplant room. Jill is now rushing up and down the corridor, stocking supplies and preparing generally for Matt's return.

"This is so exciting," she cries, dashing past us. "I knew he'd get his chance. I just knew it."

Paul, the eight-month-old in I.C.U., is struggling again tonight. As we pass the unit, we note with alarm the number of medical staff grouped around his bed. His mother, Jean, is weeping in the corridor. Totally out of character, we leave well enough alone. We can cope with no more right now.

The camp beds in the parents' lounge are surprisingly comfortable. We lie in the darkness and listen to the night sounds on the children's unit. At 1:00 a.m. Don gets up, hoping for news. Dr. Stevens is, at that very moment, hurrying down the corridor in search of us.

He tells Don that Matthew's lungs have almost been removed and the new organs should be arriving at any moment. Don also learns that, as expected, Matt is losing copious amounts of blood from the haemangioma. They're replacing it as rapidly as possible, but would like to transfuse some fresh blood too as it sometimes helps to stop severe bleeding. He's hoping that one of us may have a blood type compatible with Matt's. Unfortunately neither of us can oblige, and he hurries away to find a donor. We learn later that Dr. Stevens himself donated a pint, a practice performed occasionally by Mr. Murad and his team. *(More recently, fresh blood transfusions have been avoided in order to reduce the danger of transmissible infection — and especially HIV, the AIDS virus. New drug treatments and advances in blood component therapy are helping to reduce the problems of bleeding during surgery.)*

Don returns and relays the news to me. We're both strangely placid, almost emotionless. We know that the first major hurdle has been successfully crossed. The lungs with their hideous catastrophic disease, are gone, destined for the hospital lab, and then, probably, for a jar of formaldehyde — preserved for all time for the education of incredulous medical students.

I finally fall asleep, but awake with a start to the clamour of running feet and low, urgent voices. Some time later, the feverish activity ceases and the various footsteps depart, this time moving slowly, almost lethargically. The sounds are very different now, but one sound remains for a long, long time. There's no mistaking the anguish of a grief-stricken mother.

We sleep fitfully until 6:00 a.m. when the night sounds become morning sounds and we need to know what's happening. Jill has been in touch with the O.R.; Matt may not be on the ward for a few hours yet. Although the surgery was finished by three-thirty, he's being monitored in the recovery room until the bleeding subsides.

"Any news, Katie?" It's Clare and Charlotte, up and checking on progress. Marion Gavin and another transplant mum, Irene Newlove, arrive on the ward and they, too, want an update. There's a feeling of joy, of celebration, of miracles. The day staff start dribbling in shortly after seven.

The party gets bigger, minute by minute. Gayle's glasses are decidedly misty and Trudy beams with pride.

"I hear they closed the switchboard to Canadian calls for a while in the night," someone tells us. "Apparently it was like a zoo in there with everyone wanting to know about Matt!"

I'm suddenly reminded of the dimensions of Matthew's support group. My own family, up in Cheshire, hoping, praying and waiting for news of the night's operation. And Don's family back in Canada — clustered together, sipping hot coffee and puffing on cigarettes, all the time being positive, "thinking the good thoughts," as Don's mother would say. And I think of our friends in Tsawwassen and other parts of British Columbia. I think of our community, people to whom we are only a name, who have rallied around and helped us in every way possible. And the media. I had been so scared of them at first, so frightened to go public. What if the story were sensationalized? What if we were criticized? What if the reports were inaccurate? We need not have worried at all. The media have been consistently concerned and helpful. Keith Morgan's initial story in *The Province* brought us the plane we so desperately needed. The many reporters who have phoned in the past seven weeks have been courteous and supportive, ending their conversations with "We're all rooting for you!" or "Best of luck!" And I'm aware that their efforts have given us many unknown friends — people who, right now, may be thinking about and waiting for news of a little boy they've never even met.

At 8:00 a.m. Mr. Murad arrives on the unit. We're ushered into the nurses' office to see him. He appears fresh and rested; nothing indicates that he's spent the past eight hours in the O.R. He comes straight to the point.

"Matthew's chest was a nightmare, just as the scans predicted. We would never have been able to perform the operation without the use of laser equipment. As expected, the bleeding has been a serious problem. The new organs appear to be functioning well. The first twenty-four hours will be critical, and then we'll take it a day at a time."

How do you thank a man who has just made your child's life a possibility once more? There are no words that even come close to expressing the depth of our gratitude.

"Thank you, Mr. Murad," we say. And the big man is gone.

I savour the phone call to my mum. I imagine her drinking tea and eating toast and marmalade in the warmth of her kitchen. Waiting. Wondering. Sick with worry.

"Hello, Mum, it's me."

"Katie," she whispers, scarcely daring to draw a breath.

"The operation's over, Mum. He seems to be doing well. We've talked to Mr. Murad. The new organs are working."

A brief silence, then: "Oh, Katie, that's wonderful. Wonderful! Thank goodness." She asks a few more questions, an overwhelming burden lifting from her shoulders.

"I'll phone all the family," she promises, "and Bidie, too. Wonderful, Katie! Wonderful!"

We hurry back to Mrs. King's for some breakfast and a change of clothes. Mrs. King can hardly contain her excitement. We sip her delicious coffee and bask in the marvellous sense of relief.

By the time we return to P.S.U., Matt is already there. The ward is abuzz with staff and friends. Representatives from every stratum of hospital life are gathered outside the transplant room. Three young porters in grubby white jackets vie with one another for a turn at the window. Their faces are flushed and they laugh and banter together. They stare in wonder at the spectacle on the other side of the door. They couldn't have been more excited had Matthew been their brother.

Matt's awake and talking to the nurses. I can't see immediately which nurses are with him, for they're covered from head to toe in special protective clothing. Transplant patients must take the drug cyclosporin to reduce the risk of their bodies rejecting the new organs. It is, without a doubt, a wonder drug which has greatly increased the success rate in all kinds of transplant surgery. It does, however, alter the immune system, making the patient more susceptible to infection, so every care must be taken not to introduce bacteria. As expected, Matt is breathing with the respirator, and the trusty monitor, with its myriad of leads, is still in place. I have never, in my twelve years of nursing, seen so many IV bags attached to one patient. They hang in clusters, dripping their life-saving fluids into selected veins and arteries. His chest is covered by a wide plaster dressing, and six chest tubes, three on each side, draw off body fluid from the operative area. We tap on the window. One of the nurses, whom I now recognize as Gayle, tells Matt that we're here. He turns his head, smiles weakly and waves, giving us the "thumbs-up" sign. His skin is pink, a healthier colour than it has been for a long time. His eyes are bright and shining and he appears to be alert. Now I believe in miracles.

"Point your toes, son," Don calls through a crack in the door. People around must have thought that he'd finally flipped out, but the fear of nerve damage has plagued Don since we first realized that it was a serious possibility. Our eyes rivet on the two lumps that mark the position of his feet beneath the sheet. First one, and then the other, forms a weak point. No nerve damage! No paralysis! Thank God! Don is jubilant. We're both relieved.

Periodically throughout the day I think of a special family somewhere in the north of England. I think of their anguish at the loss of their child. I wonder if the child had been ill, maybe on life-support, and if the decision to "unplug the machines" had had to be made. Terrible, but at least with some warning. Or was the child in an accident? Alive one minute and irretrievably gone the next. Snuffed out like a candle, stamped on like a helpless insect. How shocking! How cruel! Whoever the parents are, whatever they do, we will be perpetually grateful to them. They have given us, complete strangers as we are, the most precious gift of our lives.

Later in the day Diane Kent arrives in the unit. I ask her about the possibility of thanking the donor family. The message could not be directly from us, for obvious reasons, since privacy and confidentiality are vital factors in the transplant program. She advises us to wait, to let the dust settle and see how Matt progresses. She's reluctant to say it in so many words, but should Matt die and the donor family learn of it, they would likely experience a double grief, as it were. And once is more than enough for anyone.

Later, passing through the hospital lobby, we're stopped in our tracks by excited shrieks. As we turn, Mr. and Mrs. Montez rush towards us. Mr. Montez, his eyes big as saucers, gesticulates wildly. His face is ashen. Mrs. Montez clutches at her chest and leans heavily on her husband's arm.

It's several minutes before we're able to decipher their verbal barrage. Their news is exciting indeed: organs have been found for Jose. Even as we speak, he is being prepared for the transplant. We can hardly believe it. After weeks of silence, two sets of donor organs become available within twenty-four hours. Could the TV publicity have made a difference already?

Don takes the agitated couple down to P.S.U.; he wants to prepare them somewhat for their son's return from surgery. They peer through the glass into Matthew's room and absorb the scene in grim silence.

When we return from supper, Matthew is stable and heavily sedated. He's propped up on pillows with his pal Doggy tucked under his arm. Doggy's black button eyes peer out over a green surgical mask, the ends of which are wrapped around his furry black ears. No one, it seems, is taking any chances.

Chapter Thirteen

Friday, August 15

Mr. and Mrs. Montez are beaming. She still clutches at her chest, but yesterday's torment is nowhere in evidence. Jose has come through the operation exceptionally well. Already, less than twelve hours after the transplant, he's breathing on his own. The advantage of his having gone into surgery in relatively good condition is blatantly obvious. He has drunk from a cup and is anticipating a light meal before the end of the day. He's alert and relieved. No wonder his parents are overjoyed!

Today, we're allowed to be in with Matthew. "Where's my morning hug?" Don asks, as he enters his son's sterile room for the first time. Don, like the two busy nurses who constantly monitor Matthew's progress, is gowned from head to foot, to reduce the risk of infection. Matt smiles sleepily and weakly lifts one thin arm. Don threads his head carefully through the maze of IV tubes and wires, and receives not only the hug, but a welcome kiss on the cheek too.

Matthew's internal temperature is slightly elevated, but his peripheral temperature is low. His body had to be cooled radically before surgery, and his hands, arms, legs and feet are still cold to the touch. Matt doesn't seem to notice — at least, he doesn't complain, but it gives Don an opportunity to help the nurses and to do something meaningful for his son. He fills surgical gloves with warm water and ties off the ends, making miniature hot-water bottles, which he places strategically for maximum effect. He rubs the bony legs and adjusts the heating pad. And all the time he's positive, for he well knows that attitude can affect the body's healing.

After lunch, Matt's blood gases are checked; they're found to be satisfactory, so an attempt is made to take him off the respirator. Matt is frightened to the point of panic. He turns a deathly shade of grey and is immediately reconnected to the machine. No one is too surprised. He has, after all, been relying on the respirator for the past six weeks. There's another problem too, one which is common to many heart/lung transplant recipients. During removal of the diseased lungs and heart, important nerves have to be cut, nerves that normally "tell" the brain that the lungs are functioning. Some patients are left with the eerie sensation of no longer feeling their own chest movements, and consequently have to "learn" how to breathe once again. Matt isn't prepared for this one. . . Clearly, this will be our next big challenge.

It's an eventful day in the parents' lounge. The "miracle baby," Lorenzo, is finally going home. We hug Giuseppe and Luciana, with whom we shared so much, and see them off for the airport.

Little Ben Newlove is leaving today as well. His assessment is completed and he's now on the waiting list for a heart/lung transplant. There's nothing for his family to do but return to Liverpool and wait for the call that will bring them rushing back to Harefield. We've become very fond of this pale boy. His stick-like arms and legs and bright, enquiring eyes immediately bring to mind the image of a "sparrow." His "beak" chatters constantly and, despite his medical handicap, his body is a study in perpetual motion. He's already tired of the wait for the ambulance.

"Wanna go, Mum. Let's go home. Wanna go, Mum, wanna go," he chirps. His mother, Irene, takes a book from her bag, which distracts him for all of thirty seconds.

"Wanna go, Mum. Wanna go. Let's go, Mum."

"We'll be off in a minute, Ben. Go and say goodbye to the nurses." He disappears down the corridor but is back again in minutes. "Wanna go, Mum. Wanna go. When are we leaving, Mum? Wanna go."

Irene explains, with considerable patience, that the ambulance has been delayed. "Wanna go, Mum. Wanna go. Let's go, Mum," the little bird sings on.

Irene rises purposefully from her seat. "You're right, Ben," she says, "it's just not good enough!" She heads for the parents' phone, picks up the receiver with one hand and holds the button down with the other.

"Hello? Is this the man from the ambulance?" she barks. "This is Ben Newlove's mother here. We've been waiting thirty minutes for the ambulance to pick us up! It just isn't good enough! If you don't come soon, I'm going to put syrup in your shoes and jelly in your underwear!" She pauses briefly. "That's better," she says, nodding at Ben, who's still mesmerized by his mother's audacity, his face expressing undisguised adulation. It is almost a minute before his uncontrollable jaws are in motion again.

"Wanna go, Mum. Wanna go. Let's go, Mum," he continues. Irene puts a large hand on either side of his face. "Ben! Ben! Read my lips," she commands. The little boy's gaze moves from her eyes to her mouth. "Shut up, Ben! Shut up!"

Sunday, August 17

Matt is stable again today. Thank God! I'm still in a state of happy collapse, for want of a better description. I'm very tired and nervous. I'd love the next month to be over. I want him off the respirator without having to go through the ups and downs that I know will occur. I want the period of rejection to be long gone. It'll probably start around the ninth day and last for perhaps a week. It may be mild, but it could be serious, even critical. It's definitely a hurdle. Infection, too, is an ever-present threat. In spite of all the antibiotics, his temperature is elevated — not drastically, but enough to remind us that it could be a problem. And on top of it all, I feel guilty. I'm well and my child is sick. I can enjoy a meal and he can't. I need a break and he badly needs support. Reason tells me that the guilt is unjustified, but I can't help it. I just want Matt to sleep, to know no fear, to feel no pain — and to wake up in a month with his body healed!

Don, on the other hand, is elated and positive — thank goodness he's there to take up the slack.

I go to church again. The minister asks if I'm new to the area. I tell him about the transplant and why we're here.

"How old is Matthew?" he asks.

"He'll be seven on Wednesday," I tell him, thinking of the times I've wondered if he'd make it to this birthday.

Don is waiting outside the church, having parked in readiness for a quick getaway. He's noisily revving up the engine, his face set in grim determination. It's precisely twelve-thirty when we reach Denham village and our destination, The Swan. The sign announcing roast beef dinners is out on the sidewalk again. We smile triumphantly. What a week this has been — first the transplant and now, to celebrate, the long-awaited roast beef lunch.

We inch our way through the crowd until we reach the bar. And there, right before our eyes, is a large platter of steaming, succulent roast beef, a bowl full of crisp, golden Yorkshire puddings, and a huge pan of roast potatoes. Marvellous!

"Two specials, please," Don cheerfully asks the young man behind the counter.

"Sorry, sir," he replies, "we're all out."

"Two roast beef dinners, please," Don repeats, pointing at the tempting platter.

"I'm sorry, sir, but it's spoken for. We have cold meals though. Ham or turkey?" he asks innocently.

"And what's that if it's not roast beef?" Don charges. A group close by pauses in their conversation, distracted by the red-faced "Yank."

"Those dinners are all spoken for, sir."

"By whom?"

"By people that came early, sir. They reserved it, you see."

"But what if they don't show up?" Don is incredulous.

"They're here already," stammers the youth. "They're just having a drink before lunch."

I slump into a chair and smile weakly at the woman opposite.

"We've been trying to get roast beef dinner for seven weeks now," I babble apologetically. "We thought we finally had some, but they say it's all gone."

"That's dreadful, dear," she answers politely.

"Three specials, please," someone calls from the end of the bar.

"They don't have any," Don hisses angrily. "If you don't have any, for God's sake, take down your sign."

"Two specials, please," from some new unsuspecting patrons.

"See," spits my generally affable husband, "if you don't take down the sign, I will!" A waitress hurries to remove the offending board.

"Two large glasses of white wine, please. If it's not all spoken for, that is!"

Tuesday, August 19

Tomorrow is Matt's birthday. We can hardly believe the number of cards, flowers, presents and telegrams that keep arriving. It's overwhelming.

The fourth chest drain has just been removed. Only two to go now! As with the others we play it up, enticing Matt to get better. "One day soon, you'll lose that respirator tube, son," Don tells him, "and then we can have a real hug!"

I'm still wrung out emotionally. It manifests as exhaustion. I can sit down anywhere, at any time, and be asleep in seconds. I think of Mr. Murad's advice to transplant parents. "You must be strong," he tells us. "You must be strong." I will be strong again. Give me a few days off for good behaviour, and I'll be ready to fight once more.

Don, in contrast, has energy to burn. He's almost frenzied in his need to be with his son, and spends hours rubbing Matt's spindly limbs, bringing him popsicles and playing games or reading to him.

The last two chest drains are removed shortly before we leave for the night. Steady progress, I tell myself. What more can we ask for?

Wednesday, August 20

Happy Birthday, Matthew! We made it! Seven years old today!

The night nurses stand outside Matt's door and peer by turns through the window. In spite of a long night's work, there's nothing lethargic about their rendition of "Happy Birthday." A short time later, the day shift take their turn. Fresh and rested, their chorus resounds down the P.S.U. corridor, inviting others to celebrate with them. Matthew smiles and raises a hand in acknowledgement.

Don and I arrive at 9:00 a.m. A stack of parcels is heaped in the corridor outside Matt's room.

"Can any of the presents go in to him, Trudy?" I ask.

"One or two won't hurt, but we'll have to swab them down with disinfectant."

"This one's a priority," I tell her, picking up an enormous Transformer. "It's from the readers of one of our newspapers at home, and I know the paper would like some feedback. If he's well enough in a few days, I could take a photo and send it to them." Trudy opens the door a few inches.

"Hi, Matt," she calls. "Going to be my boyfriend today?"

"No, he's not. He's my boyfriend, aren't you, Matt?" This from Gayle, anonymous beneath the transplant-room attire. The mock dispute continues for several minutes. Matt is unperturbed; he knows this game well.

It's my turn now. "Hey, sweetheart, look what the *Province* readers have sent you! Did you ever see such a humungous Transformer?" Matt's propped up in bed, resting against some pillows. He shakes his head, almost imperceptibly, from side to side. His face appears flushed, and his big blue eyes are shining.

"When you're a little better, we'll bring it in and you can play with it, OK?" The head nods in agreement. He closes his eyes and is asleep in seconds.

Later in the morning Sheila Pritchard, Matt's doctor from Vancouver, arrives with her husband, Hayden. We greet her with hugs and kisses, and shake the hand of Hayden, whom we haven't met before.

"This is wonderful," she says. "Is he still doing well? The Canadian media keep us up to date. Do you think I can go in and see him?" Sister Karen is in charge.

"Sorry, but no," she apologizes. "We can't be too careful, can we? All right?"

As a compromise, we take Sheila and Hayden around to the patio. Matt's window is slightly ajar.

"Hello, Matthew. Remember me? Dr. Pritchard, from Children's

Hospital at home?'' Matthew bites on his lip and screws up his face. Suddenly he grins and raises a hand in greeting.

"I'm in England on holiday, and wanted to come and see how you were getting on. I hear it's your birthday today. It's rather a special one, isn't it?'' Again the almost imperceptible nod. "All your friends at Children's send you lots of love and best wishes. Hurry up and get well quickly, won't you?''

"Thank you,'' he mouths and blows a kiss towards the window.

"We'll keep in touch,'' Sheila tells us. "We're so thrilled. Everyone's thrilled.''

The minister from the Harefield church pops in with a birthday card for Matt. "We'll pray for him on Sunday,'' he says. "Will that be all right?'' It most certainly will. We need all the help we can get!

"Katie, another phone call from Canada. Take it in the office if you like.'' The line crackles noisily. A voice echoes from a million miles away.

"Hello. Hello? Katie, can you hear me? It's Valerie Ward. I'm with Mr. MacInnes. We're calling from Expo, from the Telecom Canada Pavilion.'' The noise ceases temporarily. "Oh, that's better. We're wondering how Matthew is doing today?'' Then: "Good, wonderful, we're all so delighted. Give him a hug and tell him 'Happy Birthday' from us, won't you? Mr. MacInnes would like to talk to you. Bye from me for now.''

The Commissioner of Telecom Canada is an important man. My mouth feels dry and butterflies roam my abdomen. A male voice comes on the line, punctuating the intruding noise.

". . .on behalf of everyone at Expo, and especially at Telecom Canada, please give Matthew our best wishes. . .''

"Thank you Mr. MacInnes. Thank you very much.'' There's a dull ache at the back of my throat, and tears sting my eyes. I blow my nose loudly and return to Matt's room with the special message.

One friend had written, "When you return, Matthew, we'll make you Mayor or maybe even King!'' The letter had made Matt laugh.

"Do you feel like a king, fella?'' I tease.

He nods his head, grinning again.

Bidie, her husband Rob, and Judy and Dan stop by for a short visit. We chat on the grass outside Matt's window and watch the children at play in the sandbox.

". . .I've phoned everyone, lovey — Caroline, Kate, Annie and Wendy. They all send their love and will be coming to see you. . . don't throw sand, Judy, you may get it in Dan's eyes. . . they're so happy for you, lovey. We're all so happy. . .''

Vicki, one of the day nurses, has made a chocolate birthday cake. The day staff gather in the office and Vicki lights the candles. "Don, Katie, come and join us for a piece of cake. Do you think Matt can stand another round of 'Happy Birthday'?''

"Sorry you can't have cake, Matt," I tell him, when we've finished singing. "We'll have a belated party once you're well. You can make up for it then." He makes a face and settles for some fresh ice chips.

Among the stack of cards, there's one from Alice Dodd, whose handwriting has become familiar by now.

"God is thinking of you and so am I," the message reads. "Happy Birthday, Matthew."

What a wonderful day! I'll never forget it. As an added bonus, I receive a present, too: on several occasions, Matthew catches my eye and carefully mouths the words, "I'm feeling better." There's nothing I'd rather hear.

One niggling problem persists. Matt's temperature jumps to 40 degrees Celsius during the afternoon. He's started on a different antibiotic, and by evening the infection seems to be responding.

Mr. Murad stops by last thing. He checks the charts and his sleeping patient. "It looks like we may have pulled it off," he says, smiling. And with that, he is gone.

There's a new family in the parents' lounge. A tall man in a smart suit stands behind a pint-sized wheelchair. Its occupant, a girl of perhaps three or four years, appears as white as a porcelain doll. An exceedingly beautiful dark-haired woman pacifies a younger child, who is as healthy and energetic as her sibling is debilitated.

"I'll take her out to play on the swings," the father volunteers. "She's much too noisy to be in here." He tucks the kicking youngster under his arm and disappears in the direction of the patio.

"We've been waiting since February," the child's mother tells me without introduction, her lovely face showing the strain. "Six months and still no organs. Frances is getting worse by the day now. She really can't wait much longer . . ."

We exchange our stories, this woman and I, familiar with each other in minutes. I'm acutely aware of feeling superior, of having secured a colossal advantage. We are, after all, on the right side of the transplant. I know, from having stood in her shoes, that Frances's mum is aware of it too.

Matt has a sore at the base of his left nostril, where the respirator tube has been pressing. He knows that one of the anaesthetists is planning to change the tube to the other nostril later in the day, and he's most unhappy.

"I hate it," he mouths at Don, who, gowned and masked, is sitting at his side.

"Let's go for a bike ride, then," Don suggests. "That'll take your mind off things for awhile." Matthew nods and manages a grin. He's played this game before, and now it's easy for him to visualize the bike rides he used to love so much.

"OK, let's start, then," Don says. "Close your eyes and pretend we're back at home. I'm working at my desk, and you come in and ask me to go for a bike ride." He pauses so Matt can do this. "Am I too busy?" he asks, allowing Matt to take some control. Matt shakes his head, grinning broadly now. "Don't forget to put on your coat," continues Don. "Have you got your Transformer gloves? Oh, sorry. I forgot you have your new lungs now, and your circulation's better — you don't need your gloves in summer any more. OK, get your bike out of the shed . . . we're coming out of the driveway now — which way do you want to go, left or right?"

"Left," Matt whispers around the tube, his eyes still tightly shut.

"OK. We're going up the little hill towards Stephanie's house — and look at that, I don't even have to help you now; you can ride up all by yourself." Matt grins again. His concentration is absolute.

"Look, there's Stephanie and Shannon at the window. Let's give them a big wave. . . . On we go, around the corner onto Sixth Avenue, and left onto English Bluff. We're on the straight stretch now, and you're going like the wind! Even my big bike can't keep up to your BMX! Hey, wait for me!" Matt is smiling broadly now, loving every minute of his return to normal life.

"Down Fifth Avenue," Don continues, "past Andrew and Sarah's house, around the corner — and streak for home." Don turns on his Archie Bunker voice, much to the nurse's amusement: "It's for the gran' championship o' da woild, folks, and we're neck an' neck!

"It's gonna be close, but you reach the driveway just a hair ahead of me! I'm puffing and panting and out of breath. 'Let's do it again!' you say — you cruel, heartless beast!" Matt opens his eyes, which are sparkling with amusement. But Don's serious again, riding on the wave. "When the anaesthetist comes, just take a trip," he says. "Get out your bike, and ride where your spirit moves you. It'll be much easier."

"Now it's time for your exercises. What would Mrs. Merry say if she were here?" Matt attempts a few wobbly leg-ups.

"You have to get that tube out soon," Don tells him, "then you can eat tons of Chicken McNuggets, and get your strength up again." Matt tries a few toe-points, but that's all for today.

"Beth and I can dance together when I get home," he whispers.

"The sooner the better," his dad replies.

At five-thirty we leave for supper. Jill sees us peering through the window. She opens the door a couple of inches and talks to us through the gap.

"He's just waking up, since having the tube changed," she tells us. "Being off the respirator really tired him out. Apart from his temperature, he's doing OK, though."

"We'll be back after supper," I say. "I haven't been in with him yet today. It'll be my turn."

We drive a few miles to a restaurant called The Plough. I'm cross with Don on the way, for driving too fast and swinging dangerously around corners.

"What would he do if anything happened to us?" I admonish. "We've got enough problems without making more! If you can't drive any better than this, then I'll drive!"

The Plough is cool and relaxing. We order our food, then drink to our son's recovery. We talk about Matt's biggest hurdle at present.

"If only he could breathe without the respirator," I start. "I can't wait for the day he's breathing on his own. If only he hadn't been on it for so long before the transplant, this wouldn't be such a problem now!"

"No wonder he's so panicky when the respirator's off," Don continues, pinpointing our main concern. "He probably can't tell that his lungs are actually working. He can't feel them move because of the nerves having been cut, and he can't see his chest 'cause the tube's in the way." We mull this problem over throughout supper. Finally Don comes up with the answer.

"He needs a big mirror; that's what he needs!" he exclaims in a flash of inspiration. "Then he can actually see what's happening. He can see that his chest is moving!"

We both agree. It's a great idea. Tomorrow we'll find a mirror.

It's quarter past seven when we return to Harefield, having stopped twice on our way back — once to post some letters I had written, and again to buy a chocolate bar from the shop in the village.

Entering the long corridor leading to P.S.U., we see one of the surgeons from the transplant team. Mr. Mowat turns the corner and walks towards us. He raises his head, quite obviously seeing us, then abruptly turns on his heel and heads back down to the unit.

"We probably reminded him to write up a drug or something for Matt," I say, curious but unconcerned.

The corridor into P.S.U. seems oddly quiet. Only one person is around, standing in the doorway of the nurses' office and looking in our direction.

"Could you please come in for a moment?" she says, blocking our progress down the hall. I notice with alarm that Sister Sarah has been crying;

her pretty face is drawn and pale. Mr. Mowat stands in the office. He's ordinarily a serious man, but something in his demeanour makes my chest tighten. He's talking, but I can't hear most of what he's saying. I can just pick up odd words: ". . .breakdown. . . infection. . . haemorrhage. . . sorry. . ." The room is silent. We stand like four statues. I feel faint and sick. Hard as I try, there's no denying what we've just heard.

"Do you mean he's dead?" I ask, unsure that I've grasped the truth.

"Yes," they both say together. "We're sorry. We're so sorry."

I feel Don shudder beside me.

"Come," I say, taking his arm. "Let's sit down. We need to think." Sister Sarah follows us to a seat at the end of the office. She dabs at her eyes and blows her nose.

"What happened?" Don asks, fighting to maintain control.

"We think the stitches in the aorta gave way," she says. "Infection can do that, you know. It softens the area, then the stitches come apart. The team was on the floor — in the next room, in fact — but it all happened so quickly, there was nothing they could do. It was very fast," she adds comfortingly, "I'm sure he didn't suffer."

We're led into the corridor. I'm aware of faces, serious and sad, looking through windows and from doorways. Jill's coming toward us. She crumples, weeping, into Don's arms.

"He was so brave," she sobs. "We tried so hard. He waited too long. . ."

The room is silent, awfully silent. There's no respirator hissing, no monitors beeping, no rustle of nurses' uniforms as they go about their countless tasks. The steel poles with their plastic bags and tubes are gone, as are the catheter tube and chest-drain apparatus. Even the pictures and cards are gone from the walls. The room is devoid of everything. Everything — except Matthew.

He lies in his bed, covered from the chest down by his new yellow bath towel. His good friend Doggy is cradled in one arm. The bruise on his hand contrasts darkly with his pale skin and ashen face.

"He's gone," I say, referring to his spirit. "Why, anyone can see that he's no longer here."

Don kneels beside the bed and wraps his big arms round the frail, lifeless body. Tears course down his cheeks, coming to rest on Matthew's neck and face.

"You tried so hard, son," he says, "and so did we. Everyone tried so hard. If only you hadn't waited so long. If only it could have been different. . ."

Clare enters quietly and stands, weeping, at my side. She puts her arm around me. "It's so unfair," she sobs.

The corridor is deserted, except for Sister Sarah. "I've checked about his organs like you asked," she tells us, fighting back tears. "The only ones they can use are his eyes. They're coming from Moorfields early tomorrow."

Mercifully, my senses are paralysed. I feel as if I'm in a cocoon, insulated. . . drugged. I know it won't last long.

As we walk in a daze to the parking lot, we hear a familiar sound in the distance. The chopper appears over the treetops, stark and black against the evening sky.

Someone is about to have a second chance.

Epilogue

She was sitting alone in the otherwise empty chapel. An older woman, she was slight of build with curly, greying hair.

The service would be starting any minute. Even now the pall-bearers were bringing in the small coffin.

"Who is she?" Don asked my family and friends. But no one seemed to know.

She stood to greet us, this stranger, taking both my hands in her own.

"I'm Alice," she said, "Alice Dodd. I hope you don't mind me coming. I got here rather early. I've already sat through one funeral. . ."

Warmth and generosity continued to flow from people like Alice, and many others besides. . .

A Funeral Home director in Richmond who offered to fly Matt's body back to Canada — no strings or fee attached.

The representative of one of Canada's airlines who insisted on arranging our flight home — at no cost to ourselves.

The nursing administrator who wrote from Harefield, expressing their heartfelt sorrow and profound disappointment.

The members of our church who, long before we set foot on Canadian soil, had largely arranged and catered for the memorial service.

The list went on and on. . .

Harefield, I have heard, has undergone significant changes in the last four years. It is highly unlikely that "mice peek at patients from holes in the walls" any longer, for April '89 saw the completion of a beautiful new P.S.U. where seriously ill children are offered their best chance at life.

Gone also are the car headlights which once guided the helicopters in at night. A fully modern landing-pad now complements the other new additions (a large adult I.T.U. and an advanced Department of Cardiology) at the hospital. These improvements, together with the keen dedication of the Harefield staff, will help to ensure that the hospital remains a world-class leader in the development of transplant technology.

Canada's own transplant programs also have mushroomed in the last few years. Here in B.C. a multi-organ transplant unit was opened in 1988 at Vancouver General Hospital, and the paediatric programs at Children's are scheduled to start in the not-too-distant future. (Kidneys have been transplanted here since 1983.) The many advantages for transplant families to be able to stay "at home" — in familiar surroundings and with well-established support groups — are more than obvious.

I was sure, at first, that I would never recover from Matthew's death. Although we still had one treasured child, nothing could fill the agonizing void. The depth of our loss seemed unfathomable.

Fortunately for us, we found The Compassionate Friends — a support group for bereaved parents. This international organization first started in England in 1969 when a young minister, the Reverend Simon Stephens, brought two newly bereaved families together, and observed how much they could help each other.

Through T.C.F. we discovered we weren't alone in our grief nor had we been singled out for special punishment. We learned many things in those first few months: that grief is a process that must be worked "through" as opposed to "gone around" (or it will surely catch up with you somewhere down the road!); that the death of a child puts an enormous strain on the surviving family, and especially on the marriage itself; that depression, anger and guilt, and even the bizarre feelings of insanity, are all quite normal. It was reassuring indeed to know we were right on track! And we learned too, what every bereaved parent comes to know — that complete recovery isn't possible. We adapt, we change, and slowly, very slowly, we learn to move on. One year after Matthew's death, in fact on what would have been his eighth birthday, we found ourselves in a Vancouver lawyer's office, signing on the proverbial dotted line. The newborn babe we were lucky enough to be adopting lay asleep in a bassinet by my feet. Benjamin, now three years old, is a delightful bundle of energy and character. He has taken us back to the world of "Sesame Street," of sticky finger-marks on the walls, of endless outings to the park. Elizabeth, aged twelve, is in many ways maturer than her years would suggest. She is more like a parent to Ben than a sibling — theirs is a very special relationship.

At the memorial service, Laurie Gillespie spoke of Matt's love of Transformers, and of his understanding of how the toys could be changed quite simply from one form to another. Our belief is that Matthew, too, has been "transformed" and that his spirit lives on in another land — one that knows only sunshine and peace.

It is four years now since that summer of 1986 when we hoped and prayed for a miracle. Heart/lung transplants are being performed in ever-increasing numbers in more and more centres around the world. Inevitably, as with other advances in medical technology, the chance of success has greatly improved. There is still a sense of awe, almost of disbelief surrounding these most dramatic of transplants — these are the stories that make the news headlines and catch the imagination. But the truth of the matter is that many less spectacular transplants are performed quietly and without fanfare each and every day.

Corneal, skin, bone, heart valve, kidney, heart and liver transplants have now become almost routine — and with phenomenal success rates. Lung, heart/lung and pancreatic transplants are only a step behind in their process of evolution, offering hope to thousands where once there was none. The major handicap, unfortunately, for all transplant programs, still remains the same — a dearth of donor organs. Sometimes patients die while waiting. Others, like Matthew, simply grow weaker, and are unable to recover following surgery.

At this point, I am greatly indebted to Loretta Kane, Senior Transplant Coordinator with the Pacific Organ Retrieval for Transplantation (P.O.R.T.) Program for the following information on organ donation.

Transplantation offers many the hope of a new chance at life. The success rate continues to improve with the development of new surgical techniques, new anti-rejection medications and ongoing research. Unfortunately, there is a large disparity between the number of people waiting for this new chance and the actual number of organs made available each year for transplant operations.

Many people do not want to think about organ donation because (like making a will) it forces them to think about their own mortality. There are also many misconceptions regarding organ donation. Some people fear that making the decision to be a donor will somehow compromise their medical care should they find themselves involved in a life-threatening situation. This, of course, is untrue. It is only after all medical and surgical avenues have been exhausted that organ donation will be considered. Furthermore, determination of brain death is made by physicians directly involved with the care of the patient and never by any physicians who are involved in either organ retrieval or transplantation. This provides the necessary safeguards to eliminate any perception of conflict of interest.

Potential organ donors come largely from the "healthiest" section of our population. They are often people like you and I, who suddenly, without warning, are victims of road accidents or some other tragic event — and are left brain dead. When shocked, distraught family members are summoned to the hospital, the subject of organ donation is frequently left unbroached. In this situation, many health care professionals with good intent, are hesitant to discuss the topic with the family. They do not want to "upset" them in their time of grief, feeling that they have already been through enough.

This fear, however, appears to be unfounded. In response to a questionnaire, donor families indicated overwhelmingly that they were very glad to have been given the option of organ donation. In a majority of cases, the respondents also commented that their positive decision had in fact helped them considerably with their own grieving process.

The option of organ donation should be considered upon the death of every patient. Besides giving a person in end-stage organ failure a second chance at life, it also gives the grieving family a chance to have some good come out of their loss. As in Matthew's case, his family derived considerable comfort in knowing that the lives of two people were richer because of their gift of organ donation.

Many people, while in complete agreement with the transplant programs, are unaware of how to become an organ donor. In addition to signing a card (which are readily available by contacting the provincial donor agencies and motor vehicle branches), it is very important to discuss your wishes with your next of kin — as organ donation will not proceed unless their permission is obtained.

For families who have addressed this issue and who have signed their donor cards, the agony of indecision, should it ever arise, is thankfully removed.

Loretta Kane
Canadian Association of Transplantation

Canadian Organ Donor Programs

Within Canada, each region has an agency responsible for organ donor awareness. For further information, please contact:

British Columbia:
Pacific Organ Retrieval for Transplantation Program (P.O.R.T.)
855 West 12th Ave.
Heather Pavillion, D10, Room 19
Vancouver, B.C., V5Z 1M9
(604) 875-4665

Alberta:
Human Organ Procurement and Exchange Program (H.O.P.E.)
University of Alberta Hospital
8440 112th Street
Edmonton, Alberta, T6G 2B3
(403) 492-1970

Foothills General Hospital
1403 29th Street N.W.
Calgary, Alberta, T2N 2T9
(403) 283-2243

Saskatchewan:
Saskatchewan Organ Donor Program
University Hospital
Box 86, Room 315
Saskatoon, Saskatchewan, S7N 0X0
(306) 244-2323

Manitoba:
Manitoba Transplant Program
Health Sciences Centre
700 William Street, Room E421
Winnipeg, Manitoba, R3E 0Z3
(204) 787-2071

Ontario:
Central M.O.R.E.
984 Bay Street
Toronto, Ontario, M5S 2A5
(416) 921-1130

Multi-Organ Retrieval and Exchange Program (M.O.R.E.)
Toronto General Hospital
200 Elizabeth Street, BW2-630
Toronto, Ontario, M5G 2C4
(416) 340-3587

Multi-Organ Transplant Service (M.O.T.S.)
University Hospital
Box 5339, Station A, Room 4TU60
London, Ontario, N6A 5A5
(519) 663-3000

Ottawa Civic Hospital
Ottawa Civic Hospital
1053 Carling Avenue
Ottawa, Ontario, K1Y 4E9
(613) 761-4221

Ottawa General Hospital
Ottawa General Hospital
501 Smyth Road
Ottawa, Ontario, K1H 8L6
(613) 737-8498

St. Joseph's Hospital
St. Joseph's Hospital
50 Charleton Avenue
Hamilton, Ontario, L8N 4A6
(416) 522-4941

Kingston General Hospital
Kingston General Hospital
76 Stuart Street
Kingston, Ontario, K7L 2V7
(613) 548-3232

Quebec:
Metro Transplantation
Metro Transplantation
1560 Rue Sherbrooke East
Montreal, Quebec, H2L 4K8
(514) 527-0047

Hotel-Dieu de Quebec
11 Cote du Palais
Quebec City, Quebec, G1R 2J6
(418) 694-5475

Centre Hospitalier
Universitaire de Sherbrooke
375 Argyle Street
Sherbrooke, Quebec, J1J 3H5
(819) 563-5555

Nova Scotia:
Multiorgan Transplant Program
> Victoria General Hospital
> 1278 Tower Toad
> 8V-249 Transplant Unit
> Halifax, Nova Scotia, B3H 2Y9
> > (902) 428-5500

New Brunswick:
Saint John Regional Hospital
> Saint John Regional Hospital
> Post Office Box 2100
> St. John, New Brunswick, E2L 4L2
> > (506) 648-6111

Newfoundland:
Organ Procurement Exchange Network (O.P.E.N.)
> Health Science Centre
> 2443 Prince Philip Drive, Level II
> St. John's, Nfld., A1V 3V6
> > (709) 737-6600